Oby's Wisdom

A Caveman's Simple Guide
to Holistic Health and Wellness

Dr. Mark William Cochran

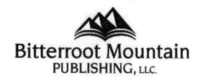

Bitterroot Mountain
PUBLISHING, LLC.

Oby's Wisdom!
A Caveman's Simple Guide to Holistic Health and Wellness

Interior design and formatting by Kimberly Martin
www.JeraPublishing.com

Cover design by Robert Craddock
www.CraddockDesign.com

Photographs of the author by Kathleen Cricket Windsong

First print edition, 2010
Second print edition, 2012

ISBN 978-0-9817874-6-6

Library of Congress Control Number: 2011941253

Quantity discounts are available on this book as an educational resource, gift, premium, bonus or other purpose. The content and design of *Oby's Wisdom* can be customized to meet your unique needs.

For information, please contact:
Bitterroot Mountain Publishing
P.O. Box 3508
Hayden, ID 83835-3508
editor@BitterrootMountainLLC.com

Oby's Generosity

Oby's Wisdom represents a fundamental shift in our approach to healing, health and healthcare—a shift away from intervention (even if it is "natural") and back toward reconnecting with the gifts of Nature.

These two wonderful nonprofit organizations share the ideals, vision and wisdom that this book offers. Because I believe in them and support them wholeheartedly, I will donate 5% of the profits from *Oby's Wisdom* to each one. Their important work benefits all of us. When we support them, we also support each other, Mother Earth and all of humanity.

Organic Consumers Association (OCA)

One of the most important factors in our individual and collective health is the food we eat. The most healthful, nutritious food available is that which is closest to Nature's design— organic and locally produced.

The Organic Consumers Association (OCA) is a 501(c)3 nonprofit organization campaigning for health, justice, and sustainability. They are the only organization in the U.S. focused exclusively on promoting the views and interests of the nation's estimated 50 million (and growing) organic and socially responsible consumers. They represent the organic, family farm, environmental, and public interest communities. The efforts of the OCA help to preserve uncompromising standards for organic and locally produced food, and expand its availability for us all.

The OCA supports our interests globally in crucial issues of food safety, industrial agriculture, genetic engineering, children's health, corporate accountability, Fair Trade, environmental sustainability and other key topics. Learn more about this important organization at: **www.OrganicConsumers.org**.

Oklahaven Children's Chiropractic Center

One of the most vital concerns of our time is the health and well-being of our children. The Oklahaven Children's Chiropractic Center is the best example I know that shows the breathtaking power of Nature to heal. Oklahaven's mission is to help sick and disabled children regain their health through a natural way of life that includes chiropractic care, whole foods, fresh air, sunlight, physical activity, and lots of love and support.

When parents bring their children to Oklahaven—often as their last hope—miracles happen. Babies hold their heads up for the first time, stop having seizures and nurse without pain. Severely challenged children learn to move independently, speak clearly without a stutter, and run and play.

Dr. Bobby Doscher, the president and CEO of Oklahaven recently told me, "The children tell the story." Dr Bobby and Oklahaven are contributing to a worldwide shift in consciousness by showing that every child can reveal the magnificent human potential that all of us *already* have within us.

Oklahaven is a 501(c)3 nonprofit organization that relies solely on the generosity of private donations without federal, state or United Way funding. Please visit their website: **www.Chiropractic4Kids.com**.

Kudos for Oby's Wisdom!

"Finalist"
—2013 Best Indie Book Awards

"Indeed this book contains a great deal of wisdom. We all need to be reminded of the age-old messages about healing and wellness, and have them presented in a way we can understand and utilize. *Oby's Wisdom* can be your guide and coach as you learn to live and love yourself and your life, and enjoy the physical benefits which go with them."

—Bernie Siegel, M.D.
Author of *365 Prescriptions For the Soul*
and *Love, Magic & Mudpies*

"To discover well-being, to honor your potential and live your unique perfection are eternal truths that one cannot help but treasure in reading this book."

—John Castagnini
Founder and Creator of ThankGodI.com

"This delightful creation of the author, my friend and colleague, Dr. Mark William Cochran, reveals the empowering truths about our choices and existence in the physical, mental, spiritual and emotional planes of life. We are all spiritual beings, having a human experience, striving to give our Innate Intelligence freedom to express itself fully and completely. The wisdom and truths revealed herein regarding the fundamental, basic principles of our existence will empower the reader to live a life of excellence and enlightenment. A MUST READ!"

—Dr. Rose Lepien
Past Chair, Parker College of Chiropractic Board of Trustees
Past President, World Congress of Women Chiropractors

"Today's wellness revolution has become a confusing forest of 'outside in' adjunctive therapies. *Oby's Wisdom* brings the clarity to allow us to see the forest through the trees. Finally, a book that brings it home: Wellness comes not from 'out there,' rather, we find it first and foremost 'in here.' As one reads *Oby's Wisdom*, the fog of confusion lifts and the reader becomes empowered. *Oby's Wisdom* is a must read for anyone invested in their health and well-being."

—Arno Burnier, D.C.
Founder and Seminar leader of Master Piece Seminars,
Café of Life, and Zeechi

"Oby's Wisdom gives us a deep insight in very clear and simple terms of how to take a closer look at our inner being. The message is ground-breaking and will genuinely change your life!"

—Dr. Sarah Farrant
Author of *The Vital Truth;*
Accessing the possibilities of unlimited health
www.DrSarahFarrant.com

"In *Oby's Wisdom*, Dr. Mark William Cochran reminds us of two simple yet oft forgotten truths: that the Universe has already given us all that we will ever want or need; and that health and well-being do not come to us, they come from within us. At times fun and light-hearted, and at others, deep and thought provoking, *Oby's Wisdom* is an important work and a delightful read."

—Guy Riekeman, D.C.
President, Life University

"I have to say that when I was first asked to read your book, I was not very enthusiastic about reading another book from a so-called 'health expert' that promises real wisdom but only delivers a new version of the same old outside-in garbage that keeps everyone in a state of learned helplessness. But I was very pleasantly surprised by *Oby's Wisdom*! Not only is your book filled with the inside-out truths people need to know, it has something for everyone! It doesn't matter whether the person is just beginning his or her journey toward wholeness or has been advancing for many years. Your book gives everyone something useful to continue their journey toward health, wellness and wholeness. From the simplest ideas about what health is and where it comes from, to specific day-to-day rituals and strategies, to very advanced thinking about the very nature of Life itself, I loved all of *Oby's Wisdom* and I will enthusiastically recommend it to everyone. Thanks for sharing it with me. It is truly an honor to call you a colleague and I know your book will help many people change their lives."

—Kevin Donka, D.C.
Chirothots

"I am inspired by the wisdom and simplicity of *Oby's Wisdom*. Dr. Mark William Cochran has an uncanny ability to remind us of the power and the beauty that resides within each of us. Mark's message is a simple, profound truth that has been lost or disregarded by most of the medical teachings of the western world. Read this book, share it with others and reconnect to the truth and the beauty of who you were meant to be. This book is a treasure trove of inspiration, wisdom, truth and simplicity."

—Jane Burnier
Life coach, teacher, speaker, mother and lover of nature

"Oby's Wisdom is a beautiful common sense approach to health, healing and life. At a time when people have access to an infinite amount of information, Dr. Mark William Cochran has provided a

straightforward and yet comprehensive approach that can be easily integrated into anyone's life. It's truly so simple, a caveman could do it."

—Sue Brown, D.C., L.C.P.
Founder and Developer of Bio-Geometric Integration
Owner of Essence Quality of Life Center

"Oby's Wisdom is an enlightening journey into the reader's potential to experience the truth that their healer is within. It allows the reader to take responsibility for their life and health. *Oby's Wisdom* inspires the reader to discover their untapped potential for health and happiness."

—Virginia Ellen
International spiritual teacher and author
Virginia appears in *What If? The Movie*,
along with other experts on emotions, the mind,
human biology and the law of attraction.

"This book is an enlightening 'quick read' with ageless wisdom deserving deep and lingered contemplation. I greatly appreciated the amalgamation of quantum physics, metaphysics and the core philosophy of chiropractic. This book truly exemplifies the principles and practices of vitalism. It is an essential read for the emerging paradigm shift of consciousness."

—Jeanne Ohm, D.C.
International Chiropractic Pediatric Association,
Executive Director
www.ICPA4Kids.org
Pathways to Family Wellness magazine, Editor in Chief
Panel Member, *Mothering* magazine, "Ask the Experts"

"*Oby's Wisdom* opens the door for you to explore the depth and breadth of the dazzling life potential that awaits, within reach, right inside of you. This fun and entertaining book will keep you smiling and turning the pages as it teaches and inspires you to reveal your genuine beautiful and perfect self."

—James A. Sinclair
Creator of *What If? The Movie*

"'*You cannot fight darkness, you must turn on light. You cannot fight disease, you must turn on life.*' This profoundly insightful book is teeming with wisdom we all once knew, but have forgotten. Through Mark, the body shares with us its remarkable intelligence and natural attraction to abundant health. Oby reminds us that wellness is more than the absence of illness or disease—wellness is conscious alignment with our life force. Whether you're concerned with dieting or vaccinating your children, or seeking a fuller sense of aliveness, this body/mind/spirit fount of simple truth will inspire you to a lifelong dance with real health. Thanks Mark, you brought me home."

—Karen Wright
Author of *The Sequoia Seed:
Remembering the Truth of Who You Are*

Table of Contents

Acknowledgements

Many people have played an intricate role in the genesis of this, my first book. I am grateful to all of you for who you are and all that you do.

A host of friends, colleagues, clients, editors, subject matter experts, booksellers and fellow writers reviewed my manuscript at various stages of development, and provided excellent feedback and insight that took *Oby's Wisdom* from a set of loosely organized thoughts to the completed book you have before you. Kathleen Cricket Windsong, M.A., Valerie Way, Susan Mitchell, Barbara McDaniel, Jane Burnier, Dr. Lynne Brett, Dr. Colleen Hathaway, Dr. Lynn Peterson, John Cochran, Ethan and Shannon Harrison, Susan Francis, Ph.D., Harvest Rich, M. L. Staats, Lisa Ernst and Nancy Harlocker, a hearty thank you to one and all.

To my fellow members of the Idaho Writers League (IWL) who critiqued my work with expertise and tact, and helped me begin to learn the ropes of the publishing world, thanks to all of you. One IWL member who deserves special appreciation is Mary L. Smith who believed in my ideas, my vision, my writing and me, and prodded me until I finally got the job done. Thanks, Mary. Your support has made a world of difference.

I am also grateful to the members of my mastermind group: Rich Hopkins, Shawna Beese-Bjurstrom, Johnny

Johnston, Harvest Rich and Jim Mohr. Many thanks to all of you for your input and guidance, and for holding me accountable for the milestones I set.

As a practitioner in the holistic healing arts, I have been blessed with some wonderful guides who have seen me through the transformation that has unfolded in my life since my days as a chiropractic student. Dr. Bobby Doscher, Dr. Arno Burnier, Jane Burnier, Dr. Sue Brown and Dr. Lynne Brett, all of you have my deepest gratitude and respect.

For the second edition of *Oby's Wisdom*, I express heartfelt appreciation to Steve and Bill Harrison and the amazing staff of their Quantum Leap program. Special thanks go to Geoffrey Berwind for his storytelling expertise, for helping me break through my self-constructed barriers (no matter how deeply I dug in my heels), for his sense of humor and for a wonderful new friendship. And to my QL accountability partners—Jamie Wolf, Mark Daugherty, Tamara Gerlach, Angela Lauria, Sharón Lynn Wyeth and Tim Wilson—another huge thank you! I look forward to continuing our friendship and mutual support for a long time to come.

My warmest, most heartfelt appreciation goes to my beautiful and loving wife, best friend and partner in all things, Kathleen Cricket Windsong. Not only has your love illuminated my life; your support, patience, energy, wisdom and insight have helped transform *Oby's Wisdom* from a very good book into a remarkable one. Your gifts are a catalyst for making me a better writer, doctor and person. You speak your wisdom with eloquence, you teach it with grace and beauty, and most importantly, you live it from your heart. Thank you for everything!

Preface

Historic Perspective

Oby, the main character in this book, is the most successful doctor in history.

The most widely accepted anthropological accounts hold that humans first appeared on Earth some 2.4 million years ago. The first medical school was founded in ancient Greece about 700 B.C. This means that, for 99.99% of human history, The Doctor Within was the only doctor available to us. This amazing doctor allowed our species to flourish and expand to the farthest reaches of the globe. Still today, The Doctor Within is the best doctor we have.

Oby the caveman, and his family and friends serve as an entertaining illustration of the powerful simplicity that Mother Nature provides all of us for pursuing a life of vibrant health, well-being, love, fulfillment and happiness. *Oby's Wisdom* is not a scholarly treatise on prehistoric humans; rather, it is my own lighthearted projection of the lives of a few fictitious cave dwellers. If some of the information seems a bit of a stretch, I ask you to enjoy it in the whimsical spirit in which I wrote the book.

The characters in *Oby's Wisdom* rise above the stereotypi-cal view of cavemen as mindless, club-wielding, knuckle-dragging brutes. In reality, later prehistoric humans were people of depth and intelligence whose lives included much more than the practical tasks required for survival.

During the Middle Paleolithic Period—also known as the Middle Stone Age—dating from 300,000 to 30,000 years ago, our ancient ancestors are known to have created art and music, followed shamanic spiritual and healing practices, lived within egalitarian social structures, engaged in long-distance trade, cared for their elderly, and conducted ritual burials. Fully developed language emerged during the more recent Upper Paleolithic Period or Late Stone Age, which extended from 50,000 to 10,000 years ago. There is even evidence that Upper Paleolithic humans may have enjoyed leisure time and sporting activity.

Health Perspective

I once heard a radio commercial paid for by a plumbers' union stating that plumbers have saved more lives than have doctors. The truth in that claim answers a question that may arise as you read this book.

Since Oby illustrates the benefits of an ancient and simple approach to health, some may point out that, in this era of modern medicine, life expectancy is higher and infant mortality lower today than in prehistoric times. Although this is true, I suggest that medical advances have played a much smaller role in preserving human life than one may think. Public health improvements such as modern plumbing, efficient waste disposal, and cleaner and safer living conditions have been far more significant than medicine in allowing you and me to enjoy longer, healthier lives. An excellent resource for learning more about this is the thoroughly researched and insightful book, *Reclaiming our Health; Exploding the Medical Myth and Embracing the Source of True Healing*, by John Robbins.

The Names Have Been Changed.

Throughout *Oby's Wisdom* I tell real life stories to illustrate important points. While maintaining the essential substance of each story, I have changed some names and personal details to assure the confidentiality of those involved.

With that, I invite you to imagine life as one of Oby's compatriots, to see the world through his eyes, and to embrace the timeless and universal lessons he has come to teach you.

Introduction

> *Keeping your body healthy is an expression of gratitude to the whole cosmos—the trees, the clouds, everything.*
> Thich Nhat Hanh

A deep sense of peace and appreciation welled up in Oby as he watched a parade of elegant clouds float past in the deepening summer twilight.

Bliss.

Obsidian J. Stone shared a life with his wife, Fern, their baby son, Scooter, and their dog, Proto, in the days when woolly mammoths roamed the plains and stone tools were state of the art. The only person who could get away with addressing him as Obsidian was his mother. To Fern and everyone else he was just Oby. His mother didn't mind when others called him Oby. In fact, it was his doting dad who bestowed the nickname upon him when he was just learning to crawl. But to his mom, he would always be Obsidian. It was such a distinguished name.

Oby made his living hunting woolly mammoths, dodging saber toothed tigers, and gathering fruit, nuts and firewood. Historical differences aside, Oby was much like you and me. At the end of a tough work day, he looked forward to going home, kicking back and letting the pressures of the day melt away. Instead of zoning out in front of the tube, Oby loved to amble up to a nearby hilltop, ease into a soft cushion of clover and take in a colorful sunset. Occasionally, Fern, little Scooter and Proto came with him. Often, he came alone. He marveled as the clouds made their majestic procession across the long misty valley and the distant snow-covered mountains beyond. Mother Nature had so many incredible gifts to offer, and her beautiful cumulus creations were among Oby's favorites. Their silent splendor moved him and he was fascinated with the important role they played in the intricate web of Nature. Oby enjoyed pondering the clouds and gazing in wonder.

Oby and his Paleolithic peers lived by a deep, profound, yet simple wisdom born of an intimacy with Nature. The cave dwellers were tuned in; they still sensed their inextricable link with Mother Earth, the heavens and Spirit. They paid attention to seasonal rhythms, weather changes, and the movements of the Earth, Sun and Moon. Their lives flowed with the natural cycles of Nature.

Take clouds, for example. To Oby, each misty monolith was beautiful and perfect in its own way. He knew that dark clouds brought rain, lightning and snow, and which cloud formations signaled a coming storm, but he never considered trying to change the clouds, control them, or make clouds of his own. He just loved each one for its own unique and important contribution to Nature. Oby saw each and every cloud as a creation of simple beauty and perfection. Oby's wisdom was the wisdom of simplicity.

The cave dwellers' way of life is long gone, but the wisdom of Nature is just as valid and important today as it ever was.

Many people never pay any attention to clouds any more except for the ones that bring rain or snow, and maybe the ones on their screen saver. The complexity of our society brings amazing levels of stress into our lives. We have forfeited our wisdom for data, education, and scientific proof. Knowledge is useful; it has made countless wonderful contributions to humanity. The flip side is that our exclusive focus on academic advances fogs our understanding of Nature and life. We have become so dependent on external authority that we have lost awareness of our *selves*. In some ways, we are no longer sentient beings.

The volume of scientific data that humanity has produced is so massive that we have trouble keeping track of it. So much of it is contradictory, and the experts are ever disagreeing with each other. Just look at the many theories about how we should eat. Years ago, books and magazine articles taught us to count calories. The next generation of experts told us: "Forget the calories; they aren't important. Keep track of your fat. Low fat is the way to go." And most recently: "Oops. We've been wrong all along. Fat is good. Carbs are the enemy. Avoid carbs like the plague."

We need calories. Always have; always will. We need fat, too. Always have; always will. Carbs? Same thing. These mixed messages can lead to confusion. And our confusion leaves us feeling powerless.

Turn Your Health Inside Out!

This is one of the most pivotal, foundational, empowering, and life changing concepts you will ever read. There are two critical elements to turning your health inside out:

1. Developing a self-affirming and empowering holistic wellness *mindset*
2. Living an enlivening holistic wellness *lifestyle*

Part One of this book will help you develop your new holistic wellness mindset; Part Two will teach you how to adopt a holistic wellness lifestyle.

Your mindset is the most crucial element of living a healthy and vibrant life. The proper mindset involves empowering your Doctor Within, that doctor who has been with you for your entire life and the wisest doctor you will ever know. Unfortunately, The Doctor Within is all too often misunderstood, neglected and even maligned in the conventional western mind.

Nature designed each and every one of us to be healthy and vibrant. Even before birth, all living beings carry a vital energy—a life force—within. The concept of a life force is a timeless and universal one. It has been a fundamental belief in the healing arts around the world for thousands of years. Anyone familiar with martial arts, traditional Chinese medicine, Reiki, Qigong or acupuncture will understand chi, qi or ki—words used in the Far East to describe life force. A central concept in the practice of yoga is prana, another word for life force. Hippocrates, the father of modern medicine, based many of his teachings on physis, the vital energy that animates all living things in Nature.

Nature gave you a physical body to allow you to express life. Pain and disease are often the result of diminished life expression. It won't come as a shock if I tell you a pattern of sleep deprivation, fast food, and sedentary habits will lead to illness. Conversely, sometimes pain can be the result of perfect life expression. For example, if you break a bone, it will hurt. The pain is a built-in protective mechanism that helps keep you from aggravating the injury. Your brilliant body is doing exactly what needs to be done. What a gift!

Your life force, directed by an inner wisdom, is what allows you to be healthy and alive. Your body is smart. You already know—innately—how to heal and be healthy without even having to think about it. Nobody has to tell you how; Nature designed you that way.

You are blessed with all of the vibrance, energy and immunity you will ever want or need. Whenever you feel a lack of energy, it is because your body is not *expressing* that energy. The same goes for immunity. You always have 100 per cent of it. The concepts of "boosting energy" or "enhancing immunity" are misguided. Vibrant health, energy and immune functioning reveal themselves as you express your inherent vitality.

No pill, therapy, herb, machine, concoction, healer, exercise, diet or anything else can give you health. That's why establishing the mindset of turning your health inside out is so critical.

Of course, if you habitually refresh yourself with a good night's sleep, enjoy your favorite physical activities, enliven your spirit through yoga, prayer or meditation, maintain a positive outlook on life, drink lots of pure water, and take pleasure in eating a balanced mix of fresh, organic foods, then you have the best chance possible of enjoying good health.

You are inherently healthy. The life you experience comes from what you think *and* what you do. A vibrant and healthy life is an outward manifestation of your physical, mental, emotional and spiritual life energy.

The Basic Truth

Oby was wise because of what he did *not* know. He never had to fret over the low cal vs. low fat vs. low carb issue. He understood certain things just because they were divine truths. They still are. Much of his wisdom was innate. That same Innate Wisdom still comes as standard equipment; you and I carry it within us for our entire lives. Most people have simply lost touch with it. A life of vibrant health emerges as you reconnect with the wisdom of Nature that pulses within you. A critical step on this journey back to self is to recognize an important divine truth that I call *The Basic Truth: You are beautiful and perfect.*

Yes, *you* are beautiful and perfect.

When I tell people that they are beautiful and perfect, a common objection is, "I'm not perfect; only God is perfect." You are a creation of God. Would you suggest that one of God's creations is anything but perfect? Any such opinion is a human judgment—nothing more. "Well then," you may ask, "aren't beauty and perfection judgments, too?" The way I see it, beauty and perfection are divine truths. The way to rise above our judgment is to acknowledge them as The Basic Truth and recognize that whenever we are unable to see the beauty and perfection in ourselves or others, it is because we are looking through human filters darkened by a lifetime of fear, conditioning, others' judgments and a multitude of other shadows.

The suffering soul hobbling down the street, bent over in pain, is beautiful and perfect, as is his athletic cousin who springs up six flights of stairs, the picture of robust health. An ailing octogenarian with a terminal disease is just as beautiful and perfect as her healthy, happy newborn great grandchild.

If you desire to live a life of vibrant health, The Basic Truth is an empowering point of departure.

Stop Avoiding and Start Living

I love bicycling. Anyone who pedals a bike has encountered a lot of bumps and hazards in the road: rocks, broken glass, potholes, sewer grates, old shopping carts (I speak from experience); you name it. Although awareness of these impediments is important, one of the most important skills I have learned for staying upright is to keep my focus on the track I want to take, and not on the obstacle. We tend to be drawn where we focus. If you rivet your gaze on the jagged pothole in the middle of the bike trail you are more likely to slam right into it. Concentrating on the path around the pothole will allow you to cruise merrily on by.

When it comes to our health, we still worry about obstacles rather than choosing to follow the smooth track. In the last couple of decades, our approach to health has evolved somewhat, but we still have not made a fundamental shift in consciousness. More and more, we seek alternatives to the invasive drugs and surgical procedures that conventional medicine has to offer, but we do so for the same old reasons— to treat disease and symptoms. We're still focusing on the potholes.

Why swerve when you can live? When life presents obstacles, relish the adventure of your journey. As Bernie Siegel, M.D. teaches us in his book, *Prescriptions for Living:* "Remember that success and healing refer to what you do with your life, not how long you avoid death."

It's Simple

Simplicity empowers. Simple wisdom was all that our fur-clad forebears ever needed. Oby never went to an urgent care clinic. Neither he nor Fern ever stuck their noses in a diet book, and they would not have bothered with a food guide pyramid even if they had one. Pharmacies and operating rooms did not exist, and Scooter never had any vaccinations. There were no health food stores where they could stock up on vitamin and herbal supplements. No one ever read any health magazines, traveled to holistic festivals or felt the need to hire a personal trainer. Yet the humans of that bygone age grew and they thrived, and they populated our entire planet.

Part One of this book is devoted cutting through the confusion and complexity of today's healthcare drama so that you can form the empowering mindset that you need to live the healthiest life you can live. Part Two will provide a simple guide to a designing a wellness lifestyle for you and your loved ones. Oby's simple guiding principles allow you to make positive, life-affirming choices by reminding you of the simple, elegant genius of Nature. Nobody gets to fill in all of the details of life but if you live, think, dream and act in a certain way, your life and health will unfold in that way.

Before we go any further, let me point out that reading this book is only one step toward better health and well-being. To get the most benefit from Oby's lessons, you need to *apply* them. So take the next key step right now. Before you move on to Chapter One, take just a moment to flip to page 187 at the end of the book. There, you will find a link where you can sign up for a free video action guide that will motivate and lead you through the most important lessons of this book.

Oby's Wisdom

- Turn your health inside out!

- Your Doctor Within is the wisest doctor you will

  ever know.

- You are beautiful and perfect.

- Yes—you—are beautiful and perfect.

- Simplicity empowers.

- On the bike trail of life, focus on the smooth path.

- Stop avoiding and start living.

- Make choices based on the simple, elegant genius

  of Nature.

Part One

The Universe Made Simple

"There is no matter as such. All matter originates and exists only by virtue of a force which brings the particles of an atom to vibration and holds this most minute solar system of the atom together... We must assume behind this force the existence of a conscious and intelligent mind. This mind is the matrix of all matter."

Max Planck
Father of Quantum Physics
From his Nobel Prize Acceptance Speech

Chapter One

Life: A Simple Concept

> *Life itself is the miracle of miracles.*
> George Bernard Shaw

So, What *is* Life?

Ah, the age old question. We are awed by life and at the same time, bewildered by it. It seems so vast and complex that its very existence can be incomprehensible. Yet life exists. We exist. You are *alive!*

One evening, when my son, Matt, was 12 years old, he and I sat down to watch a television documentary about the origins of life on Earth. The program described how certain chemical substances came into existence on the planet, thus making life possible. The documentary treated these developments as random occurrences; as though the substances just happened to bubble up from the morass and come to life by happenstance. In reality, life—in the form of life force—existed first. This life force was created by an intelligence which also crafted matter in such a way that it could express that life force.

Webster's New Collegiate Dictionary defines *Life*, in part, as: "1a. the quality that distinguishes a vital and functional being from a dead body; b. a principle or force that is considered to underlie the distinctive quality of animate beings."

Here is my own definition as it applies to health and well-being: *Life is the force of Nature inherent in all living beings that allows them to grow, thrive, evolve and creatively expand.*

Life is Intelligent

The traditional philosophy of the chiropractic profession explains life in simple terms, beginning with The Major Premise of Chiropractic: *"A Universal Intelligence is in all matter and continually gives to it all its properties and actions, thus maintaining it in existence."*

Universal Intelligence gives some matter the properties necessary for life. Examples are you, Oby, a tree and an amoeba. Some matter, such as a can of paint and a salad fork, lack the properties necessary for life. They can never be alive. Within living beings, an important component of Universal Intelligence is Innate Intelligence, which directs life force in all of the functions necessary for healing and growth.

Physical and chemical processes alone do not create life. There must be a life force to cause those processes to occur, and to orchestrate them in perfect harmony. As I sit here tapping out this manuscript, I am alive. Someday, I will die. Immediately before my death, the physiological processes of life will be working in eloquent synergy. When I die and those processes cease, my physical body will be exactly the same as a moment before. The matter remains unchanged—ever so briefly—until the decomposition process begins. When my life force departs, life will no longer exist in the context of Mark William Cochran. Of course, new microbes will begin to thrive in my body, and vibrant life will blossom in a whole new way within the elegant and brilliant plan of Nature. The difference between a citizen and a carcass, a tree and a two by four, and a steer and a steak, is in the design in which life is expressed.

The concept of life force is timeless and universal. Although it has only recently begun to creep its way into western thinking, it has been an important part of healing arts around the world for thousands of years. A name I often use for "life force," is "The Doctor Within." The Doctor Within goes by many other names: the yogic concept of *prana*; *Chi, Ki* or *Qi* in the Far East; and the ancient Greek *physis*. For a deeper understanding of the concept of life force, these terms are worth expanding upon.

Prana

Yoga has been enhancing lives for over 4000 years. Yoga is more than just the practice of coiling your limbs into pretzel-like poses; it is a deep, spiritual practice that enhances every aspect of life. The concept of Prana is an integral part of yogic philosophy and is used interchangeably to mean both "life force" and "breath." Through controlled breathing, one's life force can be guided, channeled and more fully expressed. Each yoga posture emphasizes proper breathing, and special yoga exercises called pranayama focus specifically on the breath. I have been practicing yoga since 1984 and can personally attest to its life-enriching power. Dedicated, deep yoga practice improves lives physically, mentally, emotionally and spiritually.

Chi, Qi, Ki

In 1993, when we lived in Japan, my son and I traveled with our karate sensei to Tokyo to see the Japanese National Karate Championships. As we watched, Sensei told us to observe how the martial artists were breathing. He pointed out that those whose breathing remained easy and relaxed would almost always be victorious over opponents whose breath became rapid, shallow or forced. Control of the breath allows a martial artist's ki to flow. In karate the ki-ai is a forceful expiration of the breath in the form of a loud shout, which accompanies a strike at the exact moment of impact. *Ki-ai* enables the martial artist to focus and extend ki. By extending ki, a martial artist summons the incredible internal power that we all possess. It is the ki-ai that allows flesh and bone to smash through a stack of bricks. Pause for a moment to ponder what implications this has in your own life. Even if you have no inclination to ever break a stack of bricks with your head, consider what you might be able to bring forth from inside of you by more fully expressing your life force. What untapped potential lies in wait?

Yoga and the martial arts are ways of life that are based on maximizing the expression of a person's inherent vitality. Practicing these disciplines, in essence, makes you more alive. I discuss them here to illustrate the idea that we can all connect more intimately with our inherent ability to express life.

Physis

The concept of a life force can be found in the earliest origins of western medicine. The ancient Greek concept of *physis* dates back to before the time of Hippocrates (460-355 BC), the father of modern medicine. Hippocrates believed that physis—

life force—provided the body the innate ability to cure itself of disease. He taught that symptoms of disease, and especially fever, were all expressions of physis. Interestingly, the modern term "physician" originates from the Greek term *physis*.

Innate Intelligence

In the autumn of 2000, I had the wonderful opportunity to travel to India on a chiropractic mission trip. One day during our visit, we took some time to visit a centuries-old mountain-top fortress. The fortress had a large population of monkeys who managed to tolerate the thousands of visiting tourists. Usually, that is. As I found out personally, sometimes they can become downright unfriendly. Acting like a clueless tourist, I tried to get close to a monkey to have my picture taken. It happened to be a female monkey who had a baby with her, and when I got too close, she felt threatened and attacked me. Nothing against Mama Monkey; she was doing exactly what Nature had programmed into her to protect her offspring. I knew better than to be so foolish, and I would have been wise to be more respectful of her space. Monkeys have sharp fingernails and the attack left me with several deep, bloody scratches on my forearm, not to mention a significantly elevated heart rate and just the slightest bit of shakiness. Oh yeah, and a red face, too.

If you have ever been to a zoo, you may have observed that monkeys occasionally throw their feces at each other. I knew what those sharp fingernails left behind when they gouged my flesh. So did everyone with me. My concerned colleagues quickly jumped to my aid with alcohol swabs, antibacterial towelettes, antibiotic ointment and sterile dressings.

No, thanks.

As Oby would have done, I let Nature take Her course. First, I allowed the scratches to bleed with no interference. Bleeding is a natural mechanism that flushes impurities and contaminants out of a wound. Had I immediately applied direct pressure to stop the bleeding, I would have forced foreign particles and pathogens deeper into the wound. As the blood flow began to ease, I applied some of my own saliva to the scratches. Saliva contains a protein called secretory leukocyte protease inhibitor (SLPI) which has antimicrobial, anti-inflammatory and other healing properties. (Why do you think animals lick their wounds?) When the monkey scratched me, my brilliant life force customized my saliva to the exact formula necessary to respond to that specific wound. Beyond my regular personal hygiene, I did nothing else. No antiseptic or antibiotic ointment found its way to the wound, nor did any bandage shield it. I knew that under conventional medicine, that type of wound cried out for a tetanus shot. I also knew the power of my innate healing wisdom, and I chose not to get one. Did I die of lockjaw? Obviously not. My scratches never got infected and they healed nicely with no scarring at all. My arm was able to heal because that is how Nature designed me. Nature intends for me—and you—to live a life of vibrant health.

What I described above is an example of my body's Innate Intelligence, aka The Doctor Within. The name "Innate Intelligence" suggests that our bodies have their own wisdom. We are all smart on the inside. When we are injured, it is the wisdom within, and not what we put on, that does the healing. When the monkey attacked me, my Innate Intelligence initiated my fight or flight response, and my internal functions shifted gears instantaneously. My pupils dilated to make my vision more acute. My hearing and mental ability became more focused. My blood glucose concentration increased to give me a surge of energy, and more blood flowed to my muscles to give me a burst of strength so I could jump away. The blood supply to my digestive organs decreased. Digestion was not important at that moment. I had to get outta there! Oby experienced similar changes whenever he walked around a bend and had a surprise encounter with a grizzly bear.

As soon as threats from protective primates or cranky carnivores ceased to exist, Innate Intelligence allowed both Oby and me to resume our normal mode of living. Our muscles relaxed, our hearts slowed back down and our digestive processes resumed. And in my case, after everyone was finished laughing, my beet red face gradually returned to its normal tone. Those thousands of internal functions that had so radically shifted just seconds earlier, gradually readjusted moment by moment, at exactly the right time, in precisely the right sequence. All of this happened within the space of just a few minutes and I did not even have to think about it.

Innate Intelligence also controls our internal thermostat. It causes us to shiver after a dip in a chilly northern lake and perspire on a sultry summer afternoon. Thousands of other functions sustain us—many we know about, others still invisible. We are all vast, mysterious universes unto ourselves. How many facets of life still await discovery? A dozen? Millions? Billions? Maybe more. Innate Intelligence knows all. This omnipotent awareness is involved with every minute aspect of your internal universe. Your Innate Intelligence knows more than your educated mind can even begin to imagine. In some of my lectures I lead into the discussion of Innate Intelligence by pointing out that I am a doctor, then asking for a show of hands of those who believe they know as much about the functioning of their body as I do. In adult audiences nobody ever raises their hand. When I pose this question to young school children, I can always count on a couple of class clowns to shoot their hands into the air. Immediately their classmates retort: "Nuh-uh. You do not." To the ones who raised their hands I offer kudos for being so smart. After this lead-in, adults and kids alike listen with rapt attention as I teach them about the magnificent wisdom that thrives within their bodies. The climactic moment of this lesson comes when I show a slide of the National Library of Medicine in Bethesda, Maryland. I explain that the shelves of this library contain the world's largest collection of knowledge about the human body. I then ask if anyone feels they know more about their bodies than what is found within that hallowed repository. Except for the shy ones, everybody raises their hand. Even those timid souls whose hands remain in their laps recognize the incomprehensible wonder of Innate Intelligence.

You are Completely Alive

You have as much life within you as any other human being on the planet. Many people find it hard to believe that they are completely alive, and flatly reject the idea that they are beautiful and perfect. With crossed arms and cocked eyebrows they ask: "So, if I'm so perfect—if I have all this life force inside of me—then why do I hurt? Why am I sick?"

In many of my wellness presentations, I use two pinecones to illustrate the concept. One of the pinecones is fresh and new. I marvel aloud at the natural artistry of its color and symmetry. Such a beautiful creation would add to the tasteful décor of anybody's home. The second pinecone is cracked and faded, and not nearly as attractive as the first. Most people would not consider decorating their house with it, but it sits right next to the other pinecone in front of a small fountain in my office. Grasping its top between my thumb and forefinger, I point out that the gravitational force of the earth is operating at 100%, everywhere, at all times. I then ask, "So if gravity is so perfect, why doesn't this pinecone fall to the ground?" Well, anyone can answer that; I am holding it up. In other words, my hand is interfering with gravity's ability to pull the pinecone to the ground. When I let go, the pinecone falls. Every single time. The dangling pinecone is a vivid illustration of what can happen with life force. When something interferes with the expression of our life force, we get hung up with pain and disease. When we remove the interference, we are free.

I continue the pinecone example by explaining that the pinecone is the flower of the pine tree. As the cone grows on the tree, seeds develop inside of it. When the seeds mature, the pinecone blossoms, and the seeds fall out and flutter away on the breeze. When a seed from the newer pinecone falls to the ground it will absorb water and nutrients from the soil, and radiant energy from the sun. In time it will germinate and grow into a beautiful, magnificent, vibrant pine tree.

Even as the pinecone fades and becomes brittle, the seeds retain their life force, sometimes for decades to come. In the early pages of her inspiring book, *The Sequoia Seed: Remembering the Truth of Who You Are,* Karen Wright describes how the largest form of life on our planet, the majestic Sequoia tree, starts as "a tiny seed smaller than a flake of oatmeal." She goes on to tell us, "Its egg-sized cone can lie undisturbed on the forest floor for fifty years before surrendering its seeds."

When one of the seeds finally makes its way into the soil and germinates, what happens? It will grow into a majestic Sequoia. As long as a seed has life remaining within it, it has every bit as much potential for vibrance that a seed from the newest, freshest pinecone has.

The lesson of the story is that the frailest, sickest person in the world is as completely alive as the strongest, and has the same potential to enjoy vibrant health. The only difference between the two is that the strongest person is expressing more life. Nature intended for life—your life—to be robust and vibrant.

Oby and Fern never needed such colorful explanations. They knew all of this already. Innately. So do you.

One quick memory jog...have you signed up for the free video action guide yet? If not—real quick—turn to page 187 for the link. I know you're eager to dive into Chapter Two, but this will only take a moment.

Oby's Wisdom

- You are alive!

- Your Doctor Within knows all.

- Nature intends for you to live a life of vibrant health.

- The key to vibrant health is to maximize your life expression.

Chapter Two

Health and Wellness— What Are They Really?

> *As for health, consider yourself well.*
> Henry David Thoreau

"What is health?"

When I ask that question, I usually hear answers like: "Well, health is not being sick," or, "Health is feeling good."

Is health simply the absence of disease? To help us ponder that, consider two hypothetical people, Jack and Jill. Jack feels great today. In fact, Jack pretty much always feels fantastic. He is young, active and strong, and this morning he loaded up his SUV for a kayaking trip on the Lochsa River near his home in northern Idaho. Jack is the picture of robust health. Just yesterday Jack had his annual physical and ol' Doc Goodfellow gave him a clean bill of health. "You're fit as a fiddle," smiled the good doctor as Jack hopped up off of the examination table.

But...

Unbeknownst to everyone, Jack recently started to develop a malignant brain tumor. Right now it is still so tiny that even the most modern diagnostic procedures cannot detect it. Besides, Doc Goodfellow never even bothers to look for brain tumors in people as young and healthy as Jack.

So, is Jack healthy?

Next we have Jack's big sister, Jill. She caught that nasty cold that everyone at work seems to be coming down with. She woke up feeling rotten. Jill is running a temperature of 103 degrees, she is hoarse from coughing all morning and she cannot stop sneezing. What she really can't stand is how raw her nose gets from blowing it so much. Poor Jill. She feels so lousy that when Jack stopped by to tell her the doc's good news, she could barely force a smile. "That's wonderful, Little Bro," she squeaked. *Cough, groan.* "Have a great time kayaking today."

Is Jill sick or healthy?

Consider what Jill's symptoms represent. First of all, why did Jill's body produce a fever? You may already know that. The fever was created by her immune system to inhibit the "bug" from proliferating in her body.

When your body is challenged by viruses or bacteria, they trigger chemical responses. These chemicals signal the body's temperature regulating mechanism to turn up the thermostat. Your Innate Intelligence knows to bump up the thermostat a little bit in response to a virus, and to crank it up even higher for a bacterial infection.

When you turn your internal thermostat up, your body's furnace has to kick in to raise the temperature. First, you get chills and start to shiver. Even with the rise in body temperature you feel cold because your temperature is suddenly lower than your new thermostat setting. The vigorous muscular action involved in shivering raises your body temperature, just like when you're bustin' out some big 360 flips at the skateboard park. In addition to shivering, your blood vessels constrict. This keeps more blood flow in the core of your body so that you do not lose body heat at the skin surface. Once your temperature reaches the new thermostat setting, your chills go away. Your skin will feel warm when your mother kisses your forehead to check for a fever. This is similar to the temperature in your home. When you turn the thermostat up, the furnace has to run continuously until the room reaches the new temperature. Then, as long as the temperature is the same as the thermostat setting, the furnace does not have to work as hard to maintain it.

Your newly elevated body temperature creates an environment where the microbe can no longer thrive. Once you come back into balance, your body knows to turn the thermostat back down to its normal setting. This is when the fever breaks. You start sweating and your blood vessels dilate. The dilated blood vessels cause a flushed appearance by allowing more blood to reach the skin surface to shed excess body heat. Along with fever, the sneezing, coughing and runny nose also serve important functions. They allow you to expel microorganisms and pathogens that have been killed by your immune system. Magnificent! Jill's cold symptoms are normal, healthy immune responses. Her body is doing exactly what Nature designed it to do.

Sometimes in conversation, people will lament that a friend or family member has "the bug." Usually, in an ominous, worrisome tone, they mention that the person is running a fever. "My husband is down with the flu and he's running a 103 degree fever."

My standard response is, "Cool!"

People gasp and their eyes open wide. "Cool? What do you mean cool? My poor hubby is sick." Granted, other people usually respond with sympathy, share their secrets for getting better and throw in a woeful story or two of their own.

It is cool that our bodies can give us such a wondrous gift as a cold when we need it. On the rare occasion that I catch a cold, when people ask how I am, I say, "Great!"

"What do you mean, great? You have a cold, dude."

"Yep. My immune system is helping me live in harmony with my environment. Isn't that great?"

So, back to my earlier question, "What is health?" The World Health Organization defines health as, "a state of complete physical, mental and social well-being and not merely the absence of disease or infirmity."

From my perspective, that definition falls short. Right now, Jack is on his way to playboat some big rapids with those crazy kayaking friends of his. Everybody who knows him would tell you that Jack is well. If they were aware of his brain tumor they would believe that Jack is not healthy—not really. These same people would say that today, Jill is obviously not in a state of well-being. But she is. The time has come to shift our perspective of what it means to be well. As Jack and Jill illustrate, feeling well and being well are not necessarily the same. You can feel fantastic while terminally ill, and you can feel awful because of a vigorous immune response that is helping you live a healthy life.

You are a Symphony

Classical music is one of the many types of music I love. My favorite symphony is Beethoven's Seventh—especially the second movement. A symphony is a beautiful musical composition performed by an orchestra made up of a large number of gifted musicians. These artists, with their diverse selection of instruments, play many different melodies in harmony with each other, bringing the symphony to life.

You are a symphony. More sophisticated than any orchestra, you consist of a vast array of complex systems, subsystems, organs, tissues, cells, and chemical and biomechanical processes. The adult human body is a thriving community made up of an estimated 75 trillion cells. These countless parts and processes work together to perform functions as obvious as the circulation of your blood, movement of your limbs, your thoughts and emotions, and perception of sensations such as heat and cold. They also include functions that take place on such a tiny scale that you are completely unaware of them. For example, the *Kreb's Cycle*—the cellular process that provides energy for cells to live and function—is generating energy in thousands of trillions of microscopic power plants throughout your body right now. (A thousand trillion looks like this: *1,000,000,000,000,000.*)

There are untold numbers of other functions, large and small, working in synergy in your inner universe, nonstop. For you to live—to express life—everything from the major systems all the way down to your countless intracellular processes must play in harmony. You are a wondrous and beautiful symphony.

Who conducts this magnificent symphony? Your life force. As long as your life force can express itself with no interference, you perform a harmonious and delightful symphony.

But what happens when there is interference? Let's pretend that you are the world's most gifted virtuoso violinist playing in a performance with one of the world's finest symphony orchestras. Suppose an audience member walks up onto the stage and stands in front of you, completely blocking your view of the conductor. Would you be able to play your part of the symphony? Of course you would. You are, after all, the greatest violinist in the world. You can still read your music, listen to the other musicians and play along with them. Even so, would your performance be flawless? Perhaps not; a bit of disharmony may result from the lack of communication between you and the conductor. Since you are such a gifted violinist, probably nobody but you will notice the disharmony. In other words, the life expression of the orchestra is diminished, but to such an insignificant degree that no "symptom" manifests.

Now, what if 25 more people joined the first on stage, each one blocking a different musician's view of the conductor? Will these musicians be able to play their part of the symphony? Of course they will; this is the world's finest orchestra. But will it be the orchestra's best possible performance? Probably not, because so many musicians are unable to see the conductor. Now, because of all of the interference, the disharmony may become noticeable to the audience. In other words, the expression of the orchestra has been so diminished that we now have a symptom in the symphony.

For the orchestra to come back into harmony, an important factor would be for the musicians to be able to follow the conductor's directions without the interference of the stage crashers. The first response would be an innate one—the musicians would simply shift their positions a bit so they could see the conductor. If the trespassers continued to block the musicians' view, an usher might ask them politely to leave. If they remained, then someone could call security and have them forcibly ejected from the concert hall. Once they were gone, the orchestra would be able to play beautifully again, because that is what orchestras do. The point is that the orchestra is inherently capable of restoring the harmony it lost due to the interference. Even if the source of interference is removed by external means, ultimately, the orchestra's ability to return to a state of harmony is due to the talent of the musicians and the conductor, rather than the security guards who removed the interference.

Do Germs Cause Disease?

What caused Jill's cold? Germs? Conventional science teaches us that germs are the cause of disease. Taber's Cyclopedic Medical Dictionary defines *"Germ Theory"* as, "Theory that certain diseases are the result of the presence of pathologic microorganisms in the body." The same dictionary defines *"germ"* as, "a microorganism, esp. one that causes disease."

So, do germs cause disease? To answer that, we will delve into another important and time honored theory, the Fly Theory of Garbage Dumps. The Fly Theory states: "Garbage dumps are due to the presence of the flies that buzz around them." I hope you get a good chuckle from this tongue-incheek analogy. We all know that flies do not cause garbage dumps; on the contrary, the dumps provide the environment that allows the flies to proliferate. We find flies everywhere, but large concentrations tend to exist where the environment allows them to, like at your local sanitary landfill.

Tomorrow you may go to work, school or the store, and be sneezed on by someone who has the latest bug that is going around. You may catch it, or you may not. If germs caused disease, you would catch the bug every time you were exposed to it, and so would everybody else. Germs are ever present so if germs were the cause of disease we would all be sick all of the time. To quote Bartlett Joshua Palmer, D.C., known as the Developer of Chiropractic: "If the 'germ theory of disease' were correct, there'd be no one living to believe it."

Like flies, germs are everywhere. I learned in a pathology class that the average person in one of our nation's cities will inhale 10,000 different types of viruses, bacteria and fungi every day. Right now there are more bacteria in your mouth than the number of people sharing our cozy planet. We will never be able to avoid germs; they are an inescapable part of our everyday existence. Germophobes provide a comfortable home to as many germs as Charlie Brown's hygienically challenged buddy, Pig Pen. No problem. Our immune system allows us to live in harmony with them. Germs are present in disease, but they are also prominently present in perfect health.

An article published in June 2000, in the prestigious medical journal, *The Lancet,* detailed how even some people infected with the frightening Ebola virus develop no symptoms at all. Clearly, germs do not cause disease; a disharmonious internal environment does. In Jill's case, the disharmony might have come from a stressful workplace, shivering in a drafty room, too many nights of burning the midnight oil, or living on super-sized drive-through meals.

At the beginning of this chapter I asked what health is. Here is my answer: Health is harmony.

Now another question—where does health come from? Answer: Within. You already possess vibrant health. Right now. The same goes for boundless energy and well-being.

"But wait a minute," you protest. "How can that be true? Vibrant health? Not me. I've been sick for years."

"I don't have boundless energy. I'm tired."

"Well-being? No way. I can hardly get out of bed in the morning."

Nature blessed us with all of the health, energy, vitality and well-being we will ever want or need. Energy, health and happiness come from only one place—within. You already own them. Feeling sick or tired are, in their own ways, perfect expressions of life. Each manifestation is a gift—an opportunity to go deeper inside to learn, grow and evolve.

As I said in the introduction, no pill, therapy, herb, machine, concoction, healer, exercise, diet or anything else can give you health. True—if you get a restful night's sleep, enjoy a breakfast of fresh, whole foods, get your heart pumping at a fun spinning class, and then relax with a nice, hot shower, you will feel great. Realize though, that that feeling of well-being does not come from outside of you. Your healthy habits enliven the physical, mental, emotional and spiritual aspects of your being that allow you to fully express the life force you have inside of you. Health, vitality, energy and vibrance are yours to bring forth. Always.

Lottery Tickets for Health

We are a society obsessed with miracle cures and quick fixes. *Lottery tickets!*

When it comes to financial security, some people invest their money wisely. Every month, like clockwork, they set aside a certain amount of money for the future. They know that no matter how modest their income may be, by being committed over the long term, their wealth will grow and grow and keep on growing.

Other people buy lottery tickets. They spend a few bucks a week—or sometimes a lot more—on lottery tickets, hoping for the big payoff. Money spent on lottery tickets is largely squandered. Worse yet, by depending on lottery tickets, people deny their own ability to build wealth. What if, instead of buying lottery tickets, all of that money went into a carefully thought out investment plan?

Some people invest wisely in their health by making a commitment to living a healthier lifestyle. Among the many investments they can make in their health and well-being are such pursuits as eating more fresh, whole foods; regular exercise that is fun; meditation or prayer; and practicing a living art such as yoga, tai chi or qigong. Shrewd investors engage in these healthy practices because they know they are good for the body, mind, emotions and spirit. No matter how well or ill they might feel today, by staying committed to their health over the long term, they can be sure their health investments will grow and grow and keep on growing.

Today, too many people love to buy lottery tickets for health. They take the latest new wonder drug or magical herbal concoction to cure their disease (your body already knows how to cure disease); they visit someone with a fascinating new machine that detects and "corrects" electromagnetic or energetic disturbances in the body (your body can already do that); they take miracle potions that supposedly correct chemical imbalances (your body can do that, too). Others travel to a distant land or across town to visit a healer claiming mysterious, divine healing powers. (You have been granted the same divine gift.)

Of course, all of these potions, devices and miracle healers have page after page of testimonials from people extolling the miraculous healings they have experienced. The testimonials may very well be true. Visit a lottery web site and you will probably find success stories there, too. Some people do hit the lotto, but not many. What if everyone took the time, money and energy they spent on these health lottery tickets and invested them in organic foods, yoga classes and a new basketball? Trying to hit the lotto is almost always fruitless.

I am not saying that herbs, potions, machines and gifted healers are useless. Any of them can be incorporated into a comprehensive, balanced, long term wellness strategy. Just as there are many ways to build a successful and lucrative financial investment portfolio, there are different approaches to living a wellness lifestyle. The difference between buying lottery tickets and shrewd investing is in your intention. If you perceive your only hope to be a quick and easy payoff from lottery tickets, you deny your own power and you are destined for ongoing disappointment. On the other hand, investing wisely will pay off. Trying to get well quick is the same as trying to get rich quick.

Get Out of the Way of Your Doctor Within

Drugs and natural remedies can interfere with important natural functions of the body. Earlier, we described how Jill's body produced a fever as a natural immune response to the virus that was proliferating in her body. The fever was protecting her so why take it away? But that is what many people do. As soon as a fever hits, they sprint to the medicine cabinet or

herb shelf for a remedy to bring it down. We have been condi-
tioned to look for external solutions to problems, and forget
about our inherent vitality.

Two perfect examples of this are the worldwide Severe
Acute Respiratory Syndrome (SARS) scare that occurred in
late 2002 and early 2003, and the perceived threat of an avian
flu pandemic in 2005. With all of the hype and hysteria surrounding these impending disasters, everybody missed the
most important thing: We all have an immune system.

In both instances, we read news stories about heroic public
health measures that governments instituted globally and
locally. In 2002, countries imposed severe travel restrictions
and quarantines. U.S. customs and immigration inspectors
were trained to recognize SARS symptoms and were ordered to
detain people suspected of having SARS. Scientists and doctors
shifted into high gear to try to find treatments and vaccinations for SARS.

In late 2005, we witnessed the same overreaction with dire
predications of an avian flu pandemic. In November of that
year, I wrote an article for my local newspaper entitled:
"Pandemic? Don't Panic." As part of my research for the
article, I did a Google News search for "pandemic." The
result—20,800 hits. A lengthy scan of 100 articles turned up
the same trends over and over again—drugs, quarantines and,
of course, a massive overdose of fear. New Zealand had a plan
to seal its borders, Kalamazoo was ready to take the temperature of all incoming travelers at its airport, Europe built a 677
million Euro "war chest," and of course everyone beseeched
the Pharma God for a new vaccination to deliver us from this
evil scourge. Sadly, I did not find a single article about the

natural steps we could take to stay in good health. SARS revisited.

With both SARS and the bird flu, governments and health organizations around the world appeared to ignore the most basic yet most important form of protection—our own immune systems. Nature designed us to be able to defend ourselves against disease—any disease. I am not suggesting that we are impervious to all diseases. Some present a greater risk than others, but no matter what the disease, our immune system provides the critical first line of defense. Aggressive public health measures may be helpful but if people do not have strong immune systems, those measures may prove to be almost pointless. Would a bank hire the best trained security guards and install a state of the art surveillance system...then leave their vault unlocked?

Compare our immune defense with Oby's ability to defend himself against wild animals. On any given day, Oby faced the potential of attack from a variety of different animals. He had the ability to defend himself, to some degree, from any of them. A baby three-toed sloth was no threat at all, but an attack by a grizzly bear would have been much more serious. He could never have defeated an aggressive grizzly in hand to hand combat, but there were still measures he could take to defend himself. If Oby happened to be close enough to a tall tree, he could try to escape by climbing the tree. If not, he could possibly use a large heavy stick or rocks to try to fend off the attack. If the worst case happened and he got mauled, he would have curled up, played dead and hoped to survive. In all of these cases, Oby would have had a better chance of survival if he were strong and healthy rather than weak and infirm.

The same holds true when our "attacker" is a disease. Obviously the common cold presents far less risk than Ebola, but no matter what disease we are exposed to, the first responder is the immune system. As I mentioned earlier, some people become infected with Ebola and recover without ever showing any symptoms. The reason—a strong immune response. If you come in contact with Ebola, SARS, the oh-so-scary bird flu or the common cold, you are much better off with a strong immune system. Whether you are well or feeling sick, focus first on your body's own natural potential for vibrant health.

Health comes from within and only from within. The more fully you express your life force, the healthier you will be.

Wellness

Wellness is a way. It is not an end or even a means to an end. Wellness is a way of living—a way of being.

Wellness is a popular buzz word today, but unfortunately, most people have only a fuzzy understanding of what wellness really is. I once heard a prominent physician define wellness as, "the prevention and management of disease." Doc, I respectfully disagree. Wellness is about health and vitality; it has no relation to disease.

Most people believe prevention and wellness to be the same. On the contrary, they are fundamentally different from each other. Let me illustrate the difference by using business as an analogy. Two new business school graduates, Winifred and Tanicus (Win and Tank to their friends) have just earned their MBAs and are charging out into the world of big business to make their fortunes. Tank's strategy is to steer clear of the pitfalls of the business world so that he can avoid failure. His outlook and approach are based on fear. Tank has a failure consciousness. Win, on the other hand, has chosen to achieve success. She understands what it will take to succeed, and she devotes her time, energy and resources to move in that direction. Win has a success consciousness. So, time to place your bets. Who will win and who will tank? My money is on Win to win.

What we concentrate on, we invite into our lives. Many "wellness" programs have nothing to do with wellness because, ultimately, they seek to prevent disease. They approach health from the same fear-based failure consciousness that Tank carries with him into the business world. This does not mean that prevention is bad; it certainly has its place. If it is our main focus, though, it can keep us rooted in the world of disease. A wellness perspective, on the other hand, opens the door to vibrant health, well-being and maximum expression of your vast human potential. Which would you prefer to invite into your life?

Why Live a Wellness Lifestyle?

Just because!

Enjoy healthy foods, exercise and a spiritual practice not to overcome fibromyalgia, lose thirty pounds or bring that pesky blood pressure down another 20 notches, but *just because* they are good for your health and well-being. A wellness lifestyle will help a strong, healthy person to become stronger and healthier. It is also wonderful for someone with a chronic, even terminal, illness. Wellness will not cure every sick person but it will allow everybody to live the best life they can live regardless of age or where they may fall on the health spectrum. A wellness lifestyle is important even for someone who may never be "well," as judged in conventional terms.

Wellness is a journey, not a destination. Nature guided Oby, Fern and Scooter along the wellness path because it was the only one available. Today, in the face of so many conflicting and confusing choices, the simplicity of Nature is still your best guide.

One last reminder: If you haven't signed up for Oby's free video action guide yet, please take a moment right now to flip to page 187 for the link. Reading this book will be informative and entertaining. Taking action will change your life.

Oby's Wisdom

- Health is harmony.

- Invest in health. Don't depend on lottery tickets.

- Trying to get well quick is like trying to get rich quick.

- Health comes only from within.

- Health and well-being are yours to bring forth. Always.

- Wellness is a way.

- Wellness is a path, not a destination. Wellness made simple: Follow Nature's path.

Chapter Three

IT

> *The art of medicine consists of amusing the*
> *patient while nature cures the disease.*
> Voltaire

Since Oby's time, we have made healthcare very unsimple. A significant health risk we have today that Oby never had to worry about is modern medicine. The physicians and hospitals in the United States are among the finest in the world, yet according to an article that appeared in the Journal of the American Medical Association (JAMA) in July 2000, conventional medicine kills up to 284,000 Americans every year. This makes medicine the third leading cause of death in the United States, right behind heart disease and cancer. Of those deaths, less than half result from medical error. That means that more than half of the deaths are caused by medical procedures, advice and drugs administered properly and appropriately.

We are Missing Something

The United States leads the world in medical advances and Americans spend more on healthcare than any other country— over $2 trillion in 2000. Even so, according to the same JAMA article, the United States ranks 12th out of 13 industrialized nations in quality of healthcare.

In recent years, Americans have been searching for something new and different...something better. Since 1997, people in the United States now pay more visits to alternative health-care practitioners such as chiropractors, acupuncturists and homeopaths than to medical doctors. We have thousands of natural and conventional remedies and therapies, and new ones continue to emerge. Yet, as a society, our health continues to decline. So, what are we missing?

Life!

Even though people are looking outside of the medical box, we still have not experienced a fundamental shift in thinking when it comes to our health. Today's healthcare system— conventional as well as alternative—seems to ignore health and life. Our overarching concern is disease. Today, we have countless names for the ills that befall us. In Oby's day, there was only one name: "IT." Even in these enlightened times, we can still boil most of our voluminous medical texts down to that single word. We are consumed by IT.

Fighting IT.

Finding a cure for IT.

Losing IT and keeping IT off.

"Let me kiss IT and make IT feel better."

IT cetera, IT cetera, IT cetera...

We do not have a health care system; we have a disease industry. And again, that holds true for the alternative market as much as the conventional one. We may be buying more herbs and vitamins rather than pharmaceuticals to fight our colds, but we still just worry about the cold.

What message does our disease industry constantly bombard us with? *"You have a disease."* The message comes in a variety of forms; IT has many names.

"You have the flu."

"You have an external invasion of wind with internal dampness and heat."

"You have lumbalgia due to a sacroiliac subluxation."

We maintain a narrow, rigid focus on IT. Consequently, what message do we send to ourselves? *"I have a disease."* We identify ourselves and those close to us in terms of our diseases.

"I'm diabetic."

"My child is ADHD."

"My aunt is a cancer survivor."

"I'm allergic to cats."

How do we deal with IT? First we make a diagnosis—we name IT. We give IT a label and a set of parameters so we can then fight IT.

"I'm fighting off a cold."

"He's been battling his weight for years."

"She's going to beat this thing. She's a real fighter."

The *war* on cancer.

IT dominates us. We expend vast amounts of time, energy and money to fight and defeat IT. The incredible power of life has escaped our awareness.

Here is my message to you:

You are beautiful and perfect.

Sound familiar? Remember that you are inherently healthy. Make it your aim to always bring forth your beauty and perfection to the maximum possible degree. Embrace the magnificence of life whether you are experiencing a brief, minor illness or a terminal disease.

There is More to Life than IT

Life holds so much wonder and joy beyond whatever symptoms you may feel in a given moment. Suppose you are enjoying a nice drive through a place of great beauty like Shenandoah National Park, and a bird poops on your windshield. When the poo hits, it gets your attention right away. You hit it with the wipers and some washer fluid and that may "cure" the problem, but not always. Often a stubborn remnant of the spot remains—maybe large, maybe small. When that happens, do you spend all of your time complaining about the poo? Or would you rather gaze in awe at the resplendent fall colors framing the face of Old Stony Man?

Poo or beauty—you get to choose.

My Personal Journey with IT

I know what it feels like to have your life turned *inside out*!

I know the pain and the anger. (How dare this happen to *me*?) I remember hurting so bad that it seemed it would be impossible to get out of bed in the morning. I understand the endless frustration of trying every pill, natural remedy, gizmo, healer, exercise and diet—searching for that magic cure that would finally kill the pain. I know the despair of seeing a glimmer of hope begin to shine and then fade again and again...and yet again. I have felt the gripping fear that maybe this time IT will not go away; maybe I will hurt like this for the rest of my life. I even know the agony of having a rewarding, productive and successful career go spinning down the drain— gone forever— because of IT. I have been there.

When IT first introduced itself to me—and quite rudely, I might add—I was a 23-year-old second lieutenant in the U.S. Marine Corps. I was a brave and roguishly handsome soldier of the sea, accustomed to a life of high adventure and derring-do. Like all Marines, I felt immortal.

During physical fitness training, I began to feel pain in one of my hips. At first, I barely noticed it but before very long, IT began to hurt worse and worse. Soon, the pain not only interfered with my training, IT began to affect my lifestyle as well. Professionally, I had to keep myself in top physical condition. I was an athlete, an avid scuba diver and I loved to spend time in the great outdoors. Needless to say, IT had to go.

My first course of action was one of the most commonly attempted cures in the world: MIGA—maybe it'll go away. Looking back, I'm reminded of the 70's era sitcom, *Sanford and Son*. In one episode, Fred Sanford, a cantankerous old junk yard owner, was getting late notices on his bills. Instead of addressing the problem, he kept putting the bills back in the mailbox hoping they would just magically go away. I was doing the same thing with my pain, and my "late fees" kept growing and growing.

Before too long, my mailbox was jam-packed. The pain was interfering with my life so much that it finally drove me to go in and see a doctor. After endless questions, consults with other doctors and all sorts of tests, I was diagnosed with a potentially crippling form of arthritis called ankylosing spondylitis. This was scary news and it gave rise to fear and uncertainty that I was destined to live with for years to come.

The days of pain turned into weeks, which dragged into months. After being unable to participate in physical training for several months, my commanding officer put me on notice that if I did not show a big improvement—ASAP—I would be medically discharged from the Marines. That got my attention. I loved being a Marine and the prospect of getting booted out was devastating. I understood, though. Marines have to be able to hike all night and run all day, not hobble all night and limp all day.

All along, friends had been prodding me to see a chiropractor. When I was young, my mother once told me that chiropractors were "witch doctors," so I wanted nothing to do with them. But now, with my career on the line, I relented and decided to give chiropractic a try. And it helped. A lot! Not only did it help with my pain; it also opened my mind. As my healing unfolded, I started learning more and more about alternative healing, and trying new approaches.

I began to practice Yoga. Like so many other people, I first started learning Yoga as an exercise program to help me overcome my pain. It helped with the pain but, more importantly, it was beginning to transform my life. I slowly began to gain a sense that it was doing something for me at a much deeper level than just alleviating the physical manifestations of my disease.

These were the first critical steps on what was to be a long and winding road. For years, I experienced ups and downs, flare-ups and remissions. I was a fighter and I made up my mind to defeat arthritis. I pursued an endless quest for that one *thing* that would get rid of IT once and for all.

As a Marine, the only acceptable outcome for me was victory and I launched an all-out battle against IT. I enlisted every ally I could find: conventional medicine, herbs, vitamins, chiropractic, self-hypnosis, acupuncture, books, magazine articles, past life regression, visualization exercises, green lipped mussel extract—you name it—hoping to discover that one secret weapon that would kill IT once and for all. But the harder I fought, the stronger the pain became. Pain robbed me of joy, sleep, intimacy and success. It kept me from accomplishing my mission as a Marine. Worse yet, I didn't feel I was doing a very good job as a Dad. When I would rather have been playing baseball or rollerblading with my son, I was riding my recliner, parked on ice packs.

One morning, in the middle of it all: "Here, Daddy, take my blankie." My four year old son, Matt, heard my groans and saw the deep furrows of pain that were contorting my face as I was limping out the door to go see a doctor and get some pain killers. *Again!*

Although I was touched deeply by my son's generosity, that moment was a low point for me. At the time, I was a 33 year old captain in the Marines, supposedly in the prime of my life. My job—as the Marines' Hymn proclaims—was to be one of the "first to fight for right and freedom." But for the previous 10 years, my biggest battle was the one I was fighting against my own body. As anyone who has suffered with chronic pain can tell you, the pain is much more than physical. For me, the biggest challenge was despair. Marine Corps officers are supposed to stand tall and proud, the picture of confident, capable leadership. Yet, there I was, in such a pathetic state that my four year old son felt the need to give me his most cherished possession. (Well...loan it to me, anyway.)

As time progressed, my on again, off again battle with my arthritis became a lot more on and a lot less off. Although I gave it my best, eventually I no longer measured up to the Marine Corps' rigorous physical training standards. The day I had dreaded finally arrived and the military career that I loved came to an end. I felt grief and a crushing loss of self-worth. But as I stepped forward into a new chapter in my life I also felt a sense of hope.

Chiropractic had done wonders for me. Although I had a potentially crippling disease, regular chiropractic care had allowed me to serve productively in the Marine Corps for 17 years. It had such a profound effect on me that I decided to make chiropractic my life's calling. When I left the Marines, I enrolled at Palmer College of Chiropractic in Davenport, Iowa.

When I had been a chiropractic student for a little over a year, I finally had a key revelation that changed my life. One afternoon I went to listen to a guest lecturer, Doctor Arno Burnier, who has since become a close friend and a valued mentor. One profound thought he shared that afternoon that had a powerful impact on me was, "You cannot fight darkness, you must turn on light. You cannot fight disease, you must turn on life."

Wow—that was it! Rather than fight the disease, I realized I would be better off to concentrate on enhancing my life.

Despite this new realization, within a few months, I had one of my worst flare-ups ever. I could not believe it. As a chiropractic student, I was immersed in holistic learning every day. I thought I was doing "all the right things" to stay healthy: regular chiropractic adjustments, vegan diet, daily meditation, yoga, vitamin and herbal supplements. But IT came back anyway. And this time, IT hung around for over a year. It was the longest, most painful and most debilitating flare-up I ever had. Looking back, I remember it as "the big one." Every day at school, I shuffled along like a crippled old man and was late to every class. At the time, one of my professors told me that students on campus who didn't know my name just referred to me as "the guy that limps."

This time, more than any previous time, I was angry. I felt deeper despair than I have ever felt before or since. I wanted to give up. When I fell asleep at night, I knew that I was going be in so much pain the following day that it would have been OK with me if I never woke up again. I remember sitting up in bed one morning in such pain that the thought of getting out of bed seemed just about impossible. My pain was so excruciating that I flopped back down on my pillow, looked up, and said to God, "Enough is enough. Either cure me or take me."

And, right away, I got an answer: "Cure yourself or take yourself."

"Yeah, thanks for that."

As it turned out, that was just the answer I needed to help shift my thinking. My illusions, delusions and ego were stripped away, and I became more aware of my own, wondrous, ability to heal from within. Still, this new awareness was a faint voice that was all but inaudible above the din of my pain. I remained mired in the narrow, negative, fear-based objective of fighting IT.

One afternoon, when I went to the Campus Health Center for my weekly adjustment, my student doctor, following standard clinic protocol, asked me: *On a scale from one to ten, with one being no pain at all and ten being unbearable pain, how would you rate your pain today?*

I had been answering that question with some pretty big numbers for quite awhile, but now a more enlightened perspective finally began to sink in. I decided to shift my focus from fighting to thriving.

"Sorry, I'm not going to answer that anymore," I replied. "I'm not here for my pain; I'm here for my health." My student doc raised his eyebrows as I continued, "Just adjust my spine so we can turn on life! From now on, let's focus on enhancing my health and not on fighting my disease."

I wish I could tell you that after my epiphany, the clouds parted, a divine light shone down upon me from above, and I hopped off of the adjusting table and danced out the door, free of pain forever. But that did not happen. I struggled upright and shuffled out the door just as I had come in, with a slow, painful limp. Still, in that moment, with that declaration, a faint glimmer of my divine inner light began to shine through the clouds of pain, fear and despair.

For years I had hated my body. I now realized that IT was *me*, and that, in fighting my disease, I was trying to kill part of my *self*.

Now I started to love myself—my body, my being, my mind, my spirit, my circumstances, even my pain. I learned to look at symptoms and other challenges as different expressions of life rather than judging them as wrong.

This new holistic mindset laid the foundation that led to a breathtaking healing miracle in my life. The miracle unfolded over the course of several years, but beneath my conscious awareness. Wonderful changes were happening; I just could not yet feel them physically.

In late 2005, my miracle began to reveal itself. I was coming off another intense flare-up when, one morning, I woke up and felt...different. I was still in as much pain as the day before, but I knew that something had shifted deep inside.

Over the next couple of weeks, the flare-up subsided more rapidly than any previous flare-up ever had. And this time, I sensed that I would never have another one.

A few months later, in May of 2006, I drove to the nearby city of Spokane, Washington to participate in the annual Bloomsday Run. Although it's known as the "Bloomsday Run," the majority of the 40,000 participants walk it from start to finish and I had signed up as one of the walkers. Bloomsday is a fun and festive event that I can best describe as one big running and walking party that winds its way through the streets of the Lilac City. I looked forward to it every year but my pain usually prevented me from participating. So this year, I was thrilled to be there.

As I was getting ready to step off with the walkers' group, I thought back to when I first ran Bloomsday in the late 70s when I was a college student. Back then, I could run Blooms-day from start to finish—including Doomsday Hill—no problem. So now, on a lark, I decided to see if I could jog for a short distance. I thought to myself: "Hmmm...I'm feeling pretty well. Maybe I can run an entire half mile." Then I immediately dismissed the thought as a crazy fantasy.

I took off at a comfortable jog and it felt pretty good. Before I knew it, I was jogging past the one mile marker, then the two, and I jogged nonstop until I reached he four mile marker. I walked for a short distance, and then jogged some more. When I crossed the finish line I had run over six miles of the seven and a half mile race. My eyes filled with tears of joy and gratitude. I hadn't run four miles nonstop in over 25 years, and I hadn't run *at all* in over 11 years!

Bloomsday represented a new beginning for me. I decided to take up running again and I even became a triathlete. In

2007, I ran three triathlons—including a half ironman—and my first marathon.

As I write this, at age 53, I feel healthier than ever before. I love trail running, hiking, snowboarding, kayaking and plenty of other outdoor activities.

My life has *truly* been turned inside out!

IT is a Shadow

My personal years-long search for a quick fix mirrors humanity's very same quest. We are ever seeking that silver bullet that will finally defeat IT. On your next trip to the supermarket, do a quick scan of magazine covers in the racks at the check stand. They are remarkably similar from week to week. The headlines promise new cures for the ills that befall us, whether they be colds or cancer; pounds or pimples. In contrast, have you ever seen an article about "turning your health inside out"? Nope. The hottest stories are always about new miracle drugs, magic herbs, exotic foods or space age technology to help us fight IT.

We fear IT. Fear is darkness. To our detriment, many of our health decisions come from the fearful shadows that lurk within all of us. Decisions based on fear rarely prove to be the best ones. To quote Black Elk, a great spiritual leader of the Ogallala Lakota, "...it is in the darkness of their eyes that men get lost."

Conventional medicine does not have a monopoly on fear. Many alternative practitioners also play on our fears—fear of disease and symptoms as well as fear of the big, bad medical establishment. The current controversy over vaccine safety serves as a great example. Medical doctors will admonish, "If you don't vaccinate your children, they might die." *Fear.*

Others argue: "Yeah, well, vaccines kill, too. And even if your kids don't die from their vaccines, they may be permanently damaged." *Fear.*

IT is you!

Our healthcare system—oops—our disease industry is based on IT. Well, guess what? *IT is you.* That's right. As with vibrant health, IT comes only from within. Sure, there may be external factors in play such as pathogens, trauma, poor nutrition or stress, but all of that needs to be experienced, interpreted and integrated before your body can express IT. Ultimately, IT— however IT manifests—comes from within.

When you fight IT you are only fighting yourself. So stop fighting. Find peace with yourself. That does not mean to "give up and just learn to live with IT." Just stop devoting all of your time, energy and money to your disease, pain or weight, and start paying attention to your *life.* Concern yourself with enhancing your life and maximizing your life expression. Place your priority on life, rather than IT, with your loved ones, too. *"Let me kiss you and make you feel better."*

Understanding that IT is you does not mean to blame yourself for IT, but it does allow you to take responsibility for your life. Blame anchors you in the past, leaving you with a feeling of powerlessness, whereas taking responsibility gives you strength by allowing you to shape your future.

Healthcare was much simpler for Oby and his clan than it is today. They devoted their time and energy to living rather than fighting IT.

Stop worrying so much about IT and start taking care of you.

Oby's Wisdom

- Focus on the beauty of your journey, not the bird poop on your windshield.

- You cannot fight darkness, you must turn on light. You cannot fight disease, you must turn on life.

- IT is You.

- Healthcare made simple: Stop worrying so much about IT and start taking care of you.

Chapter Four

The Matrix

> *The perfect human being is all human beings put together.*
> *It is a collective.*
> *It is all of us together that make perfection.*
> Socrates

Max Planck's quote from the first page of Part One provides a good backdrop for this chapter:

> *There is no matter as such. All matter originates and exists only by virtue of a force which brings the particles of an atom to vibration and holds this most minute solar system of the atom together... We must assume behind this force the existence of a conscious and intelligent mind.*
>
> **This mind is the matrix of all matter.**

The awesome power of human consciousness is a key ingredient in the "conscious and intelligent mind" to which Planck refers. All that we say, think, imagine and dream—individually and collectively—forms the matrix within which human life originates, grows and evolves. Our thoughts and beliefs lay the groundwork for every aspect of our lives including our health and well-being. As Bruce Lipton, Ph.D., tells us in his groundbreaking book, *The Biology of Belief:* "You can filter your life with rose-colored beliefs that will help your body grow or you can use a dark filter that turns everything black and makes your body/mind more susceptible to disease."

Here are a few striking examples of the power of human consciousness.

Placebo Effect

Few really understand the placebo effect—at least not its full depth. In fact, in March 2005, *New Scientist* magazine listed the placebo effect number one in an article entitled, "13 Things That Do Not Make Sense."

The popular notion of placebo is that it serves as a stratagem to placate someone whose disease is "all in his head." Any effect from the placebo is a matter of fooling him rather than actually curing anything. Scientists who have studied the placebo effect know that there is more to it; they understand that a person's belief can trigger a physiological response that results in a real improvement in the person's condition.

Placebos play an important role in medical research. In clinical trials, experimenters divide their subjects into two groups—an experimental group and a control group. The experimental group receives the real drug or procedure while the control group gets a placebo pill or sham procedure. The participants do not know which group they belong to. At the conclusion of the study, the two groups are compared. If the experimental group has significantly better results than the control group, then the researchers declare that the new drug or procedure "works." In virtually every clinical trial, the control group shows some degree of benefit from the placebo. An oft quoted statistic in medicine is that 30% of the participants in research studies show positive results due to placebo.

A striking example of the power of placebo came in a 2001 study published in the journal *Science* that showed placebos even benefit people with Parkinson's disease. Parkinson's symptoms result from decreased levels of a neurotransmitter called dopamine in the brain. In this study, the people receiving the placebo medication experienced improved dopamine levels similar to those taking the actual medication. Keep in mind that the people did not just think they had Parkinson's disease; they had been diagnosed with it. They did not just think they improved; they did improve. Objective scientific measurements showed increased levels of dopamine in their brains. In the control group, the placebo effect, and not the drug, caused the improvement. Simply stated, the subjects' own beliefs created their dopamine production.

How, then, do we explain placebo? Simple. It is human consciousness made manifest—a component of the matrix. This means that your own consciousness can create a beneficial physical effect regardless of what disease you may have.

Holographic Consciousness

Holographic consciousness refers to one person's thoughts and beliefs affecting others, near and far. This phenomenon is possible because the matrix is a hologram within which we are all directly and inextricably connected.

In 1988, researchers at San Francisco General Hospital conducted a fascinating study that demonstrated the power of holographic consciousness. The study investigated the effects of prayer on people in the hospital's coronary care unit. As in any clinical trial, the participants were divided into experimental and control groups but did not know which group they were in. Volunteers from outside the hospital prayed every day for the people in the experimental group. At the end of the study, those who were the subject of the prayers had better outcomes than those in the control group.

How can prayer do this? Simple. As closely linked elements of the matrix, every person's thoughts and intentions affect the lives of everyone else. This is true regardless of your spiritual beliefs. Whether you believe the matrix to be God, Allah, Wakan Tanka, The Great Spirit, Universal Intelligence, the Collective Universal Consciousness, or whatever name you choose, we all share a connection within the community of human existence. To quote John Hagelin Ph.D. from the movie, *What the Bleep Do We Know!?*, "At the deepest sub-nuclear level of our reality, you and I are literally one."

Not only does our consciousness affect our own lives and the lives of others, it can even alter the physical state of matter. One of the most fascinating books I have ever read is *Messages from Water* by Dr. Masaru Emoto. Dr. Emoto, a doctor of Alternative Medicine in Japan photographed frozen water crystals under a variety of conditions. The photographs I find most intriguing are those that depict the effect of words, thoughts and prayers on the structure of the frozen crystals. In some of the experiments, jars of distilled water were left overnight with different words taped to the containers. The following day, Dr Emoto froze droplets of water from the different samples and then photographed the resulting crystals. Uplifting words such as "thank you" and "love" formed beautiful, six-pointed crystals. Harsh words like "you fool" and "you make me sick/I will kill you," rendered grotesque structures that did not even resemble crystals. One remarkable result is that the frozen crystals sometimes formed images depicting the words they were exposed to. One crystal from "You make me sick/I want to kill you," shows a figure that resembles a person with a gun. A crystal from the sample exposed to the word, "soul" has a heart in the center.

One set of Dr. Emoto's photographs was taken of frozen crystals of tap water in Kobe three days after a major earthquake in 1995. Reflecting the horror and misery of the population, the resulting structure was quite chilling. As described by Dr. Emoto, "It was a picture that made people shudder." Three months later, after an outpouring of sympathy and support from the rest of the world, and with hope replacing fear and sorrow, new photographs showed beautiful crystals.

In another experiment, Dr. Emoto set a cup of tap water from Tokyo on his desk. He sent letters to 500 former students asking them to simultaneously send "chi and soul of love" to the water, along with the wish that the water become clean. The pictures of the water prior to the good wishes showed jagged, fragmented structures. After the former students projected their thoughts of life, love and purity, the crystals became attractive, flower-like formations.

Your thoughts affect the structure of water; and your body is 70% water. With that in mind, ask yourself: How is my internal dialogue affecting me today?

Quantum Physics

Another remarkable example of how human consciousness can affect matter is the behavior of the *quantum* in physics experiments. Other words for quantum are electron and photon. Physicists consider the quantum to be the basic building block of the universe.

The quantum sometimes acts as a wave and sometimes as a particle. The two have distinctly different properties and behaviors. A particle is a distinct physical structure whereas a wave is—well—a wave. The question, then, is: When is a quantum a particle, and when is it a wave? The answer may depend on whether or not anybody happens to be looking at it. In his thought provoking book, *The Holographic Universe*, Michael Talbot describes how some physicists believe that the physical state of the quantum is determined by whether or not it is being observed. When physicists are looking at the quantum, it is a particle. When no one is observing it, experimental data suggest that the quantum is a wave. If we are looking for an electron we get an electron. If not, we don't. Even at the subatomic level of existence, what we look for, we find.

Pause for a moment to consider the implications of all of this on our health. As of 2011, the United States spends 2.8 trillion dollars each year on researching, diagnosing and fighting disease. That's 2.8 trillion dollars' worth of disease consciousness that we weave into our matrix each year.

With such a pervasive disease consciousness, can it be a surprise that medicine has become the third leading killer of

Americans each year? The fact that so many people die from medicine is not medicine's fault. Our own collective consciousness drags us into that abyss.

In his book, *Awakening to Zero Point,* Gregg Braden says: "Your thoughts are the tool that you use to bring yourself into resonance with various aspects of creation. Thoughts and feelings are your tuning mechanisms."

The time has come to bring ourselves into resonance with our nature as beings of beauty and perfection, and to tune in to vitality, love and peace. Consciously choose these as the golden fibers you weave into the matrix.

Our *Real* Reality

I sometimes hear woeful complaints such as: "Get real. Beauty, perfection, love, peace, yeah, yeah, yeah. They may make us feel all warm and fuzzy when we talk about them, but they're not reality—at least not in my world. I'm sick. I hurt. I sure don't feel beautiful and perfect. And as far as love and peace—time for a reality check. There are still too many people out there who aren't loving or peaceful. My boss is a jerk, traffic is a bitch, the bills are piling up and I have a million things to do with no time to do them. I'm totally stressed out and I'm too frazzled to go out and sprinkle love and peace upon humanity. To be honest, there isn't a whole lot of beauty and perfection in my life."

I'll grant you, that paints an accurate picture of many people's lives. And, although the details have changed over time, there have been people who have experienced life this way from as far back as Oby's time. Let me offer a more positive and empowering way of looking at life: Our day-to-day problems, stresses, aches, pains and illnesses may get much of our attention, but they are not reality. These vicissitudes of life merely cast shadows over reality, making it more difficult to see. Our *real* reality is our core essence—love, peace and vibrant health.

If you take the sickest, angriest, most violent person in the world and start illuminating layers of darkness with love, compassion, nutritious foods, plenty of fresh water, joyful physical activities, laughter, and daily meditation, who will emerge? Will we be dealing with a sicker and meaner person? Of course not. As time passes, we will come to know an ever healthier, more peaceful and more loving person. Reality— love, peace and vibrant health—will always shine through.

This point is beautifully illustrated in the powerful and in- spiring film, *What If? The Movie.* Early in the film, its creator, James A. Sinclair says, "Who we really are is perfect light, perfect happiness, perfect joy..." Throughout the movie, many other brilliant teachers expand our horizons with fascinating perspectives and compelling real-life examples of the breath- taking human potential that resides within all of us.

Visualize Your Reality

As a dedicated yoga practitioner, I am flexible and limber, and my practice includes some challenging advanced poses. During my journey with arthritis, when I experienced pain and stiffness, I sometimes found even the most basic postures too painful to attempt. Even then, I always affirmed to myself that the pain-free contortions were my reality, and the periods of limitation were opportunities for growth. When I was in pain, I still practiced as best I could while visualizing myself holding the postures as if I were completely free of symptoms. Then, as now, visualizing my reality helps me see through the shadows of perceived reality and find my way back to myself.

Just Love

> *I think I have discovered the highest good. It is love. This*
> *principle stands at the center of the cosmos.*
> Dr. Martin Luther King Jr.

Our truest, deepest, most fundamental nature is love. *Just love.* Note that I didn't say "unconditional" love. As beautiful as unconditional love may be, we can go even deeper. The term, "unconditional," implies that there can be conditions placed on love. Where conditions exist, love cannot.

Oby, Fern and Scooter had a happy little dog named Proto. They had never known a dog happier and more loving than Proto. At night, he loved to curl up next to his best friend in the world, Scooter. In the mornings, as soon as everyone began stirring, Proto made the rounds, tail wagging, wishing everyone a cheery good morning with about a hundred little doggie kisses. The love that Proto expressed was deeper than unconditional love. Proto was never even aware of the possibility of placing conditions on love. His love was the purest love of all—*just love.*

The core of your core essence—your real reality—is just love. Love is the real world.

Oby's Wisdom

- The mind is the matrix of all matter.

- Your thoughts, dreams and words are the fibers you use to weave the fabric of your life.

- The real world is love, peace and vitality.

- Reality made simple: Your deepest, truest nature is just love.

- Love is the real world.

Chapter Five

Turn Your Health Inside Out

> *You cannot fight darkness, you must turn on light. You cannot fight disease, you must turn on life.*
> Arno Burnier, D.C.

This chapter brings you to a turning point—your opportunity to make a fundamental shift in your approach to health. Here, we reframe our collective and individual understanding of health and healthcare.

Our current frame of reference: "Uh oh. Something's wrong; gotta fix it." Our primary approach to healthcare is *intervention*. This is true not only in conventional medicine, but in alternative healthcare as well.

"Uh oh. Got a cold. I'd better go see Doc Goodfellow and get some meds."

Or...

"Uh oh. Got a cold. I'd better run down to the health food store and stock up on vitamin C, echinacea and golden seal."

Taking herbs and vitamins may seem to be a more enlightened approach than taking drugs, but in most cases, the consciousness is still the same—intervention—taking something to get rid of something. I am generally a much bigger fan of natural remedies than drugs, but in terms of intention, a pill is a pill whether an herb or a drug. Pills are an attitude. Their purpose is to fight darkness.

Our new frame: "Turn your health inside out."

"I've got a cold. Cool. I love what my Doctor Within is doing for me right now. What an incredible gift! Maybe my body is telling me to take a look at how I've been treating myself. Have I paid enough attention to turning my health inside out?"

Is intervention appropriate sometimes? Of course it is—sometimes. If someone sustains an injury in a serious accident, an emergency room can be a godsend. Even so, intervention should not to be our first approach to our health.

Before I go any further, let me make it clear that I am not saying that herbs, vitamins and other natural approaches are always intervention. Any healing art—including conventional medicine—can be used either as an intervention or to turn your health inside out. The difference between turning your health inside out and intervention is in the intention. If your goal is to cure, fight or prevent a disease, you are intervening. If the intention is to most fully and outwardly express your inherent vitality, regardless of the presence or absence of disease, then you are turning your health inside out.

We Have Strayed

Today, we often reduce even nutrition to just another form of intervention. I once had a conversation with a gentleman I will call Sidney, who was telling me he was struggling with high cholesterol. When I asked about the foods he ate, Sid's response was, "I tried diet and it didn't work."

Didn't work? How far have we strayed when we look at healthy foods as an intervention that failed? Did Sid conscientiously adopt healthier eating habits? And for how long? My guess is that he made a half-hearted attempt for only a short time. Even if he made wiser eating choices for a year or two and his cholesterol levels never decreased significantly, how much would his overall health have improved? And how much better would his body be equipped to adapt to the challenges that his high cholesterol may present? Now carry that out even further. If our good friend Sid stayed with more natural, whole foods, what would his health and life look like in 5...10...50 years? In that light, even if a specific problem never goes away, good nutrition always works.

Contrast Sid's attitude with that of a woman I had spoken to a few weeks earlier. I will call her Dianna. Dianna told me that several years prior, she and her husband were self-employed and did not have any health insurance. She told me that she and her family were healthier during that period than they have been before or since. Her words were: "We've never been so healthy. Knowing how expensive healthcare is, we really took care of ourselves." They turned their health inside out. Dianna went on to tell me that now that she and her husband are both employed, they have health insurance and they know that if anyone in the family ever gets sick, they can run to the doctor for a prescription. As a consequence, Dianna admitted, they are not nearly as health conscious as before—and not quite as healthy.

Just Say No to Drugs?

War against drugs? Let's be realistic. Our society loves drugs. Watch any TV show or thumb through any magazine and you will see drug ad after drug ad after drug ad...happy people...a quick and easy cure for every problem.

One of today's hottest political issues is, which candidate is going to buy us the most drugs? *("Why should we have to pay for them ourselves? We <u>need</u> them. Getting sick isn't our fault and there's nothing we can do about it.")*

An American Family

"Sure had a tough time getting going this morning. That caffeine jolt always helps. I took little Sally to the doctor to get some antibiotics for her ear infection and made sure she's up to date on her shots. The doc gave us a couple of free samples of Tylenol, too. Wasn't that nice? That reminds me; the school nurse told me that I need to take Jimmy to the doc within a couple of weeks to renew his Ritalin prescription. Dad doesn't go anywhere without his Motrin—he calls it his 'vitamin M'—and thank goodness for his little blue buddies. (Wink.) Mom's got a big new bottle of Prozac and a few other prescriptions—not sure how many or what they're for. She probably ought to get one of those handy boxes that Granny and Gramps each have with all of the little compartments to help them keep track of which drugs to take, and when. Gee, Aunt Sarah looks great since she got Botox, doesn't she? Junior, here's the new zit cream you wanted, and I got you some cold medicine, too. I heard you sniffle a couple of times this morning. This one will help you sleep better tonight. Tomorrow morning, take this other one; it's the kind that keeps you from getting drowsy. Huh? Oh yeah...be right with you...soon as I pour

myself a glass of wine...rough day at work. OK, what were we going to talk about? Oh yeah. Just say no to drugs."

What's the real message?

Intervention Interferes

Healing is a natural process, not an event or a goal. Intervention often interrupts the process. Anyone who has ever had a cast on a broken bone knows how much their limb deteriorates while in the cast. The deterioration is because the dynamic life process is being choked off by immobility. Broken bones in casts will actually heal more slowly than if they are not casted. We cast a broken limb to stabilize the break and protect the limb from excessive motion and impact that could aggravate the injury. We do this despite the fact that we have a built-in mechanism—pain—to protect us. No one who breaks his arm this morning is going to rush off to play in a rugby game this afternoon.

Intervention can interfere with the emotional healing process as well. For example, if a person loses someone close to them, grief follows. Grief is a healing process that carries many physiological and emotional symptoms such as loss of appetite and sleeplessness. Of course, there are plenty of drugs and natural remedies available to counteract all of these symptoms and allow someone to feel more "normal." But the symptoms are all part of the mental, emotional, spiritual and physiological process of adjusting to the profound life changes taking place. Interfering with those mechanisms slows the healing process.

Often, we intervene as a reflex when it is not necessary. Take a sprained ankle, for example. When we sprain an ankle, what happens? First we follow Nature's plan, guided by our response to the pain. We limp or hop around a bit before we flop down and start rubbing it and wiggling it. We are doing what we innately know we need to do to begin stimulating our healing response. Within seconds the ankle begins to swell, and it hurts a lot—natural splinting and protection. The edema brings chemicals to the injury that are necessary to begin the healing process. The healing process is beginning to unfold with beautiful precision. Then what do we do? First we pop a few ibuprofens and ice the injury to relieve the pain and swelling. This may make us feel better, but it also diminishes the protective pain response and removes the natural splint. Then we have to wrap it with a compression bandage to protect and splint it. In so doing, we replace effective, natural protective mechanisms with second rate substitutes. We deprive our injury of the perfect, custom designed package of healing magic that Innate Intelligence rushed to the site courtesy of EdEx (Edema Express).

I am not hinting that you should never have a cast put on a broken bone. When I was in college, I once sustained five breaks in two bones in my hand. I wore a cast for six weeks because the orthopedist told me to. Trust me, if I ever have an injury like that again, the cast is going on...again. But now, with my ability to listen to my body, if I felt after two, three or four weeks that it was time for the cast to come off, I'd bring that up with the doctor.

It is not up to me to suggest that no one ever take medication for symptoms associated with grief or anything else. Intervention can be a gift, when appropriate. The decision as to when and when not to intervene is a personal one. Make that decision with the understanding of the difference between intervention and turning health inside out. Even when you intervene, you can still remain focused on turning your health inside out.

If you twist your ankle while shooting hoops in your driveway, the best tack to take may be to limp into the living room, kick back in your recliner, pop in that new DVD and let Nature take Her course. And be grateful for the pain and swelling.

That is what Oby would have done. Well, except for the DVD. On the other hand, if you twist your ankle on a rock while you are backpacking up in the Cucamonga Wilderness, it may not be a bad idea to wrap it to minimize the possibility of aggravating the injury on the steep hike back down to the trailhead.

Weigh the pros and cons of intervention with an understanding that the intervention is not what causes healing. Healing comes from within. You must decide what is right for *you* based on the factors that exist in your life.

Turning Health Inside Out

> *Consciousness is the basis of all life*
> *and the field of all possibilities.*
> *Its nature is to expand and unfold its full potential.*
> *The impulse to evolve is thus inherent in the very nature of life.*
> Maharishi Mahesh Yogi

Turning health inside out is a consciousness. More than just a way of thinking, it is a new way of being. For most in our society, this is an entirely new approach to life and health. When we shift from intervention to turning health inside out, we empower ourselves. Turning health inside out expands our possibilities and allows our natural potential to reveal itself.

Understanding the concept of turning health inside out simplifies healthcare. This new frame of reference empowers us to decide when intervention may be appropriate for us and when to leave well enough alone. I have already used the example of a cold being "cool." People who know me understand that. It is not uncommon when someone comes into my office with a cold to smile and say: "Hey, I have a cold. Isn't that cool?" To which I generally reply: "Congratulations on your cold. Now let's turn on some life."

The point is, intervention is not always necessary. Your Doctor Within is always on call to help maintain a state of balance, harmony and health just as an airplane is aerodynamically designed to maintain straight and level flight without input from its pilot. When Marine Corps and Navy pilots go to flight school, the first airplane they fly is a T-34C. My brother, John, a skilled and daring aviator who flew for the Marines for many years, describes it as "a docile, forgiving airplane." That is why they put new pilots in it. When I was a Naval ROTC student, a Navy flight instructor came to our campus to recruit pilots. He flew in with a T-34C to offer a little bit of "stick time" to his hot prospects. At the time, I was considering becoming a Marine Corps aviator (they wear cool shades) so I was one of the lucky ones who got to fly with him. This was no leisurely sightseeing excursion. After he took us through an adrenaline-pumping series of aerobatic maneuvers, his voice crackled in my headset: "You have the aircraft."

Stick time!

To demonstrate the stability of the T-34C, he had me stall the airplane. Stalling an airplane is different from stalling a car. A stall when flying means that the plane does not have enough airspeed to fly. The engine is still humming right along; you are just falling out of the sky. The pilot had me throttle back to stall speed then pull all the way back on the stick. That brought the nose up and caused the plane to veer to the side and fall, spinning, toward the earth. One moment I was cruising along, admiring the rolling green contours of Idaho's fertile Palouse Prairie; the next, I was plummeting toward it. The image of a red barn spinning up toward me is permanently emblazoned in my memory. Before we did this maneuver, the pilot had instructed me to hold the stick all the way back for a couple of seconds after the stall, then to let go. When I released my white knuckled grip after...oh...1.3 seconds or so, we eased out of the spin back into level flight. I didn't have to do anything. That wonderful airplane did it all by itself. Innately. No intervention necessary.

Of course, recovering from a spin often requires more than just letting go of the controls. Pilots train exhaustively in different recovery techniques so that they can instinctively use them if it becomes necessary. The point is, sometimes intervention is necessary and sometimes it isn't.

You are a sleek, shiny and sturdy airplane, precisely engineered for smooth, level and exhilarating flight. Often, you can get back on track just by letting yourself fly as designed. Even if you do decide to intervene, ultimately, it is your perfect aerodynamic design that keeps you winging gracefully among the clouds.

The Underlying Cause?

Today, practitioners in many healing arts see "treating the underlying cause" of our symptoms as the wise, enlightened approach to healthcare. I have a different perspective: Treating the cause is no different from treating symptoms. They are both the same—treating IT. Even the deepest underlying causes that we can perceive with our educated mind may still exist at a relatively superficial level. I will agree that it can be useful to look beneath the surface for hidden issues that, when addressed and released, can help us heal. As we discover and clear these issues, though, it helps to keep in mind that we are creations of unfathomable depth and complexity. The totality of our existence is an intricate web of spiritual, emotional, mental and physical aspects—and maybe even some dimensions that we have not yet discovered—all giving rise to infinite possibilities. Our intellect is probably incapable of grasping every underlying cause of all other underlying causes of the countless layers of deeper underlying causes of many possible outlying causes, as they may relate to all of the conceivable overlying causes...

For example, people diagnosed with depression often have chemical imbalances that their physicians believe are an underlying cause of the depression. Yes, these chemical imbalances do exist; and yes, they do correlate with symptoms of depression. And, yes, treating the chemical imbalances with drugs can "correct" the perceived imbalance and relieve the symptoms. But merely relieving the symptoms does not bring about healing. In fact, it may very well deprive someone of the opportunity for the deep, core healing that their depression is presenting them. Can we ever really know what caused the chemical imbalance in the first place? Was it a self-limiting belief? Might it have been a past trauma from childhood...or from a past life...or a future life...or one or more parallel existences? Or is it, perhaps, a karmic life lesson playing out at a vibrational level? Or...?

Most of us have seen nesting dolls—those large, rounded, hollow toy figures that you open to reveal an identical, but somewhat smaller figure. Within the smaller figure you find another smaller one, then an even smaller one, and yet another, and so on. Think of a human being as a set of nesting dolls that goes from an infinitely large doll down to an infinitely small doll, and with dolls that go not only from large to small, but also from side to side, forward and backward in time, and back and forth through every dimension and possibility. Trying to reduce symptoms and disease to a finite set of underlying causes is an oversimplification that limits the possibilities available to us on our healing journey.

As complex and incomprehensible as human existence may be, it is still useful for us to have an intellectual framework within which to make decisions about life and health. I suggest that, rather than limiting ourselves to trying to find and treat a specific cause for our problems, we spend more time and energy on fully expressing the beautiful and perfect life force that shines within each of us. We better serve ourselves when our primary approach to health and well-being is to *turn our health inside out!*

First, Turn Your Health Inside Out

Earlier, I mentioned that in the fall of 2000, I had the opportunity to travel to India on a chiropractic mission trip. While there, I picked up an intestinal parasite called giardia. Giardia has about a two-week incubation period so I felt fine while we were in India. It was not until we got home that I started to feel sick. Then it nailed me. I cannot remember ever getting so sick, so fast, in my entire life. I had terrible diarrhea and was unable to hold down anything I ate or drank—even water. It was frightening. I figured out what I had, and I decided that I was going to have to intervene. My first course of action was driven by fear. I went to a medical doctor who prescribed a course of antibiotics. After I completed the course of antibiotics, they had relieved my symptoms to a great degree, but not completely.

As I pulled myself away from the fear, I realized that I had not followed the path that I recommend to everybody else—to focus first on turning my health inside out. At this point, although I still felt I needed some sort of intervention, the next thing I did was go to my chiropractor to have my spine adjusted. I had no expectation that the adjustment, by itself, was going to rid my body of the giardia, but I also understood that if I wanted an intervention to be most effective, my body needed to be expressing life as fully as possible. Then, after my adjustment, I went to a homeopath who provided me a remedy that got rid of the giardia within a few days. In the process, I learned an important lesson. When I allowed fear to divert my focus away from turning my health inside out, my desired outcome eluded me. Only after I turned my health inside out was I able to move through the challenge that faced me.

The Decision

Early in my journey with IT, I grew to believe that I should never have to resort to conventional medical care. After all, I reasoned, those drugs have dangerous side effects. On those occasions when the pain was bad enough that I decided to take medication, I felt that I had failed. I would look at myself contemptuously in the mirror and sneer, "you drug addict." Not a great self-image, was it?

For someone who favors turning health inside out, the decision to resort to an intervention can be a difficult one, accompanied by guilt and a sense of failure. But deciding to intervene does not mean you have failed. Intervention can be a gift. Just make the decision from the perspective of turning your health inside out first. Sometimes intervention is the appropriate course of action. Once you have made your decision, trust that it is perfect for you in that moment. Whether drugs, surgery, chemotherapy, hypnosis, a homeo-pathic remedy or herbs; welcome the intervention with love and gratitude. Weave into your matrix thoughts of empower-ment and possibility rather than fear of side effects and complications.

Integrating the Past

Within our physical bodies we have vast, untapped stores of life force waiting to be released—life, ready to be turned on. These stores are in the form of previous input of energy and information that the body is holding onto but has not yet integrated. Energy input occurs in all aspects of our lives—physical, mental, emotional and spiritual—and includes input that we judge positive as well as negative. Examples:

1. *Physical* (lack of exercise, too much exercise, injury, illness, surgery, prescription drugs, alcohol, junk food, nutritional supplements, too much food, smoking, pol-lution, toxic exposure, etc.),
2. *Mental* (learning a new job, studying for a big exam, lack of intellectual stimulation, hooking up and pro-gramming your new DVD, etc.),

3. *Emotional* (new love, bringing a baby into the world, worry, anxiety, anger, rejection, deadlines, loss of a loved one, relationship challenges, etc.) or

4. *Spiritual* (not having a spiritual practice in your life, feeling that you are a victim of circumstances, seeing yourself as separate from—or lower than—the Divine, etc.).

All of the various forms of energy we are exposed to must be processed and integrated physically, mentally, emotionally and spiritually. When you experience input that you are unable to integrate, it has nowhere to go, and your body stores it. Your body can hang onto it long after the event has passed—even for the rest of your life. Chiropractors, massage therapists and other healing practitioners are familiar with the concept of the body holding onto past experiences. I remember commenting to a client of mine that she was carrying a lot of tension in her neck and right trapezius muscle. She remarked, "Yeah, that's my mother." This stored energy is a portion of your life force that is "locked up." The life force is still there, but you are not using it productively.

"Negative" energy input is commonly referred to as "stress." In our society, the predominant view of stress is that it is bad—something to be avoided or managed. Along with this belief, people generally acknowledge that some stress is "good" stress. In reality, stress is energy, and energy is neutral. It does not care whether it causes good things to happen, or bad. How this energy affects your body is determined by how it is processed.

Electricity flowing through efficient circuitry brings light, comfort and even luxury to your home. The same electricity buzzing its way through old, worn, overloaded wiring may spark a fire that can burn your house down. Hopefully the wiring in your home is routed through a good set of circuit breakers. If so, an overloaded circuit will trip a circuit breaker thereby saving your house from a fiery fate. Still, the lights will go out in part of your house. The life force in your house is still there—100 per cent of it—but part of it is blocked in the circuit breaker panel.

Input of energy is a necessary and inextricable part of our human experience. For the most part, we can handle it; Nature designed our bodies to process and adapt to most of the unending stream of energy that flows through our lives. If you are physically fit, a regular program of weightlifting (physical stress) will keep your muscles strong and well-toned. But if someone who hasn't been physically active for years charges into the gym and does the same two hour workout that he did as a high school football player, that is a surge of input that his body is no longer wired for and will most likely result in injury. After his stressed joints heal and his muscle soreness fades away, the excessive energy input from his ill-fated overzealousness may still not be integrated; he could still be hanging on to it at a deep vibrational level. In your home, you can rewire a short circuit but your air conditioner will not work until you go out to the garage and flip the tripped circuit breaker back on. Stress does not come only from traumatic incidents like overdoing it in the weight room. It can also be the result of seemingly minor but long term behaviors such as slouching in front of your computer all day or a double shot of espresso every morning. One day of slouching or an occasional cup of coffee won't hurt you but, over time, either of these behaviors is likely to diminish your life expression.

Your body has the inherent ability to process and integrate stored energy. When you do so, locked-up life force is released and becomes available for your body to use productively. Stored energy comes from events that have come and gone, either from earlier today or earlier in your life. Suppose that on the way to work today, another driver cut you off and almost ran you into a ditch. Not only did it scare you; you also got mad. You escaped physical injury, but felt traumatized by the event. The surge of fear and adrenaline from the near miss overloaded your circuits, popped a couple of breakers and, as a result, you have been shaky, tense and short tempered all day long. As you walk out of the office after a tough workday, you have a headache and an upset stomach. Then you hop into your comfortable automobile, play some of your favorite tunes and head down the road. Ahhhh. You start to unwind. When you walk in your front door, you are greeted with a kiss and a long, affectionate hug from your significant other, and the wagging tail of your loyal canine companion. You have a delicious meal, and then you relax. Maybe you read, listen to music, spend time on your hobby or play with your kids. By the time you crawl into bed, you feel much better. Your body has processed at least some of the emotion from this morning's frightening near miss and the pressure you felt all day at work. Turning health inside out can be a simple matter of integrating energy input.

A term from Physics 101 that is synonymous with "stored energy" is *potential energy*—energy that is waiting to do work. Some energy stores are necessary, but an excessive amount of stored energy in the body can be unhealthy. Conversely, processing and integrating the stored energy, and thereby restoring the smooth flow of life force, can improve your health. This is easy to understand when you consider one particular source of energy—food. One way your body processes food is by digesting it, storing it as fat then burning the fat to create energy. As long as you maintain an appropriate level of body fat, it contributes to good health and well-being. When anybody carries around too much of this unused energy source, it can cause all sorts of health problems. When you become more physically active and start burning off the fat—processing the excess stored energy—then your health improves.

The same holds true for any energy that you have not yet processed. Once your body processes it, the potential energy is free to flow and help you grow, evolve and expand.

A certain amount of stored stress can enhance a person's life, or cause problems. For example, after months of training, nervous energy can help an athlete win...or choke. If an athlete has mastered relaxation techniques, she can direct her nervous energy to her big race and excel. Physical and mental stresses have become a powerful ally. If not, her nervousness is likely to hurt her performance. The important thing to remember is that the benefits of stored energy result from a dynamic cycle of storage, use and replenishment. Energy is not meant to just sit there.

The Café of Life

The name of my first healing practice was The Café of Life, part of a worldwide movement created by Arno Burnier, D.C., a leader and visionary in the field of natural health. The Café of Life is a group of passionate chiropractors who share a common philosophy. At a Café of Life, healing comes from the heart. Then, as now, I seek to build synergistic relationships with people to help them reveal, from within themselves, lives of vibrance and vitality. My approach is to help people maximize their own, natural potential for vibrant health regardless of whether symptoms happen to be present.

When people come to one of my offices, they step into a warm, welcoming and peaceful environment rather than the atmosphere of a clinic. When you come to me for care, you will find soft lighting and an eclectic mix of beautiful art, stunning landscape photography and a variety of treasures from around the world. What I always seek to offer is a peaceful healing sanctuary.

Although I no longer call my private practice the Café of Life, my approach to healing remains the same: to turn health inside out rather than to intervene. Some may argue that when I adjust someone's spine, I am intervening to correct a problem. But remember, turning health inside out is a consciousness. Whether or not any healing act is an intervention depends on the shared intention of the practitioner and the recipient. Some chiropractors, including me, serve with the intention of releasing potential rather than correcting problems. Each time we adjust, we facilitate the expression of life. We find this to be a positive, empowering and powerful approach. To quote Doctor Sue Brown, a brilliant and visionary chiropractor:

In much the same way as the Chinese character for crisis is opportunity; every bit of tension stored in the body is a great source of potential energy, waiting to be released. The greater the tension, the greater the unhealed event, the greater the source of potential energy and healing. Each time an adjustment is given, a little bit of potential energy is released, increasing the flow of life in the body. I no longer see it as "boy you have a lot of tension," but rather, "boy you have a lot of potential." Potential to heal, potential to grow, potential to feel, potential to evolve.

When a practitioner and recipient are in agreement, this is a beautiful way to facilitate healing in any person regardless of their age or state of health. It serves thriving newborn babies, people who limp through the day in pain from an acute injury, those debilitated by chronic disease, as well as world class athletes.

Turning health inside out works with every aspect of life—body, mind, emotions and spirit. The most important component of healing is spiritual and it is an integral part of my healing approach. The spiritual importance of chiropractic dates back to the earliest days of the profession. Daniel David Palmer, D.C., known as the Founder of Chiropractic, is noted for his quote, "Chiropractic unites man the spiritual with man the physical."

Healing arts around the world have recognized the spiritual significance of the spine for thousands of years. Spiritual disciplines such as Zen meditation, yoga and the martial arts all stress proper alignment of the spine. The seven chakras (energy centers) in the body are all in alignment with the pelvis, spine and cranium. In *Autobiography of a Yogi*, Paramahansa Yogananda states, "In deep meditation, the first experience of Spirit is on the altar of the spine, and then in the brain." In my healing work, I am not only aligning the vertebrae, but bringing body, mind, emotions and spirit into alignment with each other, and with the external environment.

Healing Occurs at Different Levels

One afternoon, Oby stretched out on his back in the fragrant summer clover atop his solitary vista. Gazing at the sky, he noticed that the clouds at different levels were moving in different directions. The big, puffy ones closest to Earth floated majestically toward the distant mountains. The flat ones, higher up, raced off toward the long rolling prairie. The highest clouds he could see—the thin, wispy ones that reminded him of Fern's long, fine hair—seemed to be standing still. The waves of grass on the prairie below flowed in yet a different direction. Oby had noticed this many times before and it was pretty easy to figure out. The wind blew in different directions at different altitudes.

Crisscrossing clouds demonstrate one of the mysteries of the healing process. Your body, feelings, thoughts and spirit perform a wondrous concert of healing and growth throughout your life. Sometimes you can see cumulus, stratus and cirrus clouds all at the same time. At other times, the sun shines brightly in a sky clear and blue from horizon to horizon. On the rainiest days you can only see the lowest level, the cumulus clouds. Even when you cannot see past the rain, every atmospheric level is alive with activity.

In your body, pain and other symptoms are your first cloud layer. If they get all of your attention, they can obscure the life that still thrives beneath your misery. As the healing process unfolds, it is easy to make the mistake of believing that if you are not feeling better, nothing is happening. Just because you may not notice a change in symptoms, try not to make the mistake of believing that your chosen healing approach is not working, because *you* are working. Remember—behind the darkest, stormiest, most foreboding clouds, a brilliant sun continues to warm and brighten your inner world.

People call me a healer but the truth is that I have never healed anybody of anything. I am a facilitator, a conduit, a portal. The only one who can heal you is you. A beautiful quote to illustrate this point is from Cricket Windsong, my loving wife, and a wonderful healing facilitator: "The openness to heal can only come from within—to be receptive to the healing light available in all existence—all exists within ourselves."

As a healing facilitator, I can open the blinds in a dark room to let the sunshine in, but I did not create the sun. The healing work I offer releases the light and life that glows, endlessly, within you. Your Innate Intelligence knows where best to shine the light. You might feel better right away or it may take awhile. Regardless of what happens with your symptoms, you are healing. It is none of my business how your body's Innate Wisdom chooses to direct your life force. The process is yours and yours alone, and I have no attachment to the outcome. At first that might sound uncaring, but realize that a predicted outcome is a judgment. Nonattachment is the most caring approach of all because it honors your unique, beautiful and perfect healing journey.

Bless the Pain

A year before I graduated chiropractic college, I attended a chiropractic training camp where, for six intensive days, I was challenged to the breadth and depth of my physical, mental, emotional and spiritual being. I did some serious inner work. On the first day of the program, I read a quote in the seminar booklet, "Bless the pain for it will bear its perfect fruit in perfect time." At the time, I happened to be in a lot of pain and

I thought that was one of the most ridiculous ideas I had ever read. I wondered how pain could ever bear fruit. Up until that moment, I had judged that pain had only robbed me of my previous career, sidelined me from enjoying the activities I loved, slowed me down in everything I did and thrown my life into turmoil. For years, I only wanted to be rid of my pain so I could have my old life back.

I have since come to learn that meeting the challenge of chronic pain can be a catalyst for a beautiful creative expansion in one's life. The word, "heal" comes from the Old English word, "hal," which means "whole." Healing is so much more than overcoming pain, injury or disease. Healing is a continuing, lifelong process of growth and transformation—of becoming whole.

The pain I experienced over the years led to profound personal growth, discovery and spiritual evolution. At times I was only cognizant of the dark rain clouds in my life, while at deeper levels, I was transforming. It took me a long time to realize it but behind the pain, I was changing, growing and becoming more than what I was before. Many people experience this.

In his book, *It's Not About the Bike. My Journey Back to Life,* Lance Armstrong chronicles how his experience with cancer led him to start The Lance Armstrong Foundation. Cancer showed Lance that his human potential was much greater than winning bike races. He wanted to become an empowering voice to let others know that the disease did not have to be a death sentence. In his words, "It could be a route to a second life, an inner life, a better life." I identified with that passage so strongly that it caused me to look up and say, "Right on!" Although Lance and I have never met, I have felt a kinship with him ever since. Even though our respective experiences with IT were different, the outcome was similar. The fear and the pain caused something to spring forth from deep within—something powerful, beautiful and important.

Today, I feel I am more whole, centered and integrated than in years past. I have gained clarity as to my purpose in life and, most importantly, my focus has become, *what can I contribute to humanity?* My journey with pain is what led me here. I don't enjoy pain any more than anyone else does, but I now recognize and embrace its gifts. I am able to share these contemplations on love, peace, and wholeness because pain helped illuminate them in my life. My pain has borne its perfect fruit in the perfect time.

The Big Idea

Turning health inside out is about potential, not problems. Maximizing your potential creates an ever-expanding ripple of empowerment that reaches far beyond you. In my profession, we call this *The Big Idea*. When you transform your own life, you are illuminating the matrix and helping others transform theirs.

Several years back, a man named Michael came to see me because a friend of his had told him how much chiropractic had helped her with stress. Mike was experiencing extremely high levels of stress in his life and was hoping that I could help him cope with it. Mike is a gifted luthier; he builds magnificent guitars. After his first few sessions with me, he told me that they were wonderful for helping him deal with the stress in his life, but the effect carried him far beyond that. He said that the "supporting of life" he was experiencing led to greater clarity in his life and was helping him reach more of his potential in his work making guitars. He is able to build better guitars and, as a result, new doors have opened for him. Before, he made guitars for local musicians and students. Now, he also crafts them for college music professors and well-known performing artists, and he has caught the attention of some of the world's top classical guitarists. Turning health inside out has led to substantial, tangible improvements in Mike's life and that of his family. He enjoys better health and increased income, and his star is rising in his profession. Mike's increased potential has touched your life and mine, too. Many musicians are playing better guitars today than they were before. The world is enjoying more beautiful music. Isn't it amazing how far a little bit of increased life expression can reach?

We are all artists, working in synergy, co-creating the glorious work of art that is our collective human experience. We each have our own unique, important and beautiful contribution to offer. To quote my friend, Doctor Cheryl Berry: "Imagine that we are individual cells in this organism called Humanity. What function do you serve? What is your piece in this masterpiece?"

That is a pretty heady thought. No one among us has a clue as to what our final answer will be. Avoid the limiting mindset of judging what your potential should be, or predicting what it will be. Just maximize it...by turning your health inside out. Not even the most insightful clairvoyant can predict all of the wondrous adventures that await you. B. J. Palmer simplified it with this far-reaching insight: "It is better to light one candle than to curse the darkness. Get the idea; all else follows."

OK, time to land this spaceship. We have been floating around in the lofty galaxy of philosophy; now we need to return to the reality of Planet Earth. With so much to ponder and contemplate, remember this one critical point: Turning health inside out follows the simplicity of Nature.

Mother Nature designed us to live healthy, vibrant lives, and She provided all that we need. If She had made it too hard, we would never have survived. Oby, Fern and Scooter didn't have to follow any special procedures to turn their health inside out. They turned their health inside out all day long by being in harmony with themselves and the world around them. They did it innately, without ever having to think about it. Life had a beautiful simplicity. Today, science, technology and the complexities of our society have caused us to lose our sense of connection with the Earth and the heavens. Part Two of this book will help you to reconnect with the simplicity and power of Nature's perfect plan.

Oby's Wisdom

- Healthcare simplified: First, turn your health inside out.

- Turning health inside out is a consciousness, a way of being.

- Healing is a lifelong process of growth and transformation.

- Turning health inside out is about potential, not problems.

- Maximize your potential without trying to judge or predict it.

- Turning health inside out is just reconnecting with the simple, elegant genius of Nature.

Part Two

Turn Your Health Inside Out!
Oby's Simple Guide to
Holistic Health and Wellness

"I need no inspiration other than Nature's. She has never failed me yet. She mystifies me, bewilders me, sends me into ecstasies. Beside God's handiwork, does not Man's fade into insignificance?"

Mahatma Gandhi

Chapter Six

Spirit, Soul, Love and Healing

> *You are not a human being in search of a spiritual experience.*
> *You are a spiritual being immersed in a human experience.*
> Teilhard de Chardin

Let's pause briefly...

Before you continue reading, put the book down and take a few moments to reconnect with yourself. Close your eyes, wrap your arms around yourself in a warm, loving embrace, and say: "I just love myself. I just love *me*." Even if you have not felt that way for awhile, the love is there—right inside—waiting to resurface. Your core essence of love never stops shining. Use this time to reconnect. Pause for a few minutes and enjoy the feeling of the pure love you feel for yourself—the love that you *are*. OK, go ahead.

Wait a minute...really...take this opportunity to express love for yourself. Say it. Feel it. This can be a powerful experience for you.

Welcome back.

Connecting with your spiritual essence is the most important aspect of health, well-being and life. You are a spiritual being on a thrilling adventure in a physical body. Spirit transcends, permeates and underlies everything. Spirit is love, so at your very core, you are love. *Just* love. Remember, love is the real world.

You are a uniquely beautiful and perfect expression of the Divine. As you travel your spiritual path, you reveal your beauty and perfection—to the world and to yourself. Each adventure on your journey can reconnect you with the Divine and bring more of you to light. The most beautiful person you can be is you, expressing your beauty and perfection, and offering yourself and others the divine gifts that have been entrusted to you to share. An inspiring quote that illustrates this point was written by Bernie Siegel, M.D., in his wonderful book, *Peace, Love and Healing*: "God gave us all certain gifts, but it is up to us to decide how to use them in such a way that even the Being who gave them to us will look down one day in admiration and say, 'Hmmm, I never thought of it that way before.'"

Spirit and Soul

Concepts of spirit and soul differ widely, so it is important for me to describe the concepts as I use them in this book. I do not mean to suggest that my view is the one and only "truth."

What I offer in the following paragraphs is my present-day sense rather than a rigid, permanent set of beliefs. My spiritual philosophy has evolved—and continues to evolve—through years of living, loving, meditating, reading, writing, thinking, teaching, healing myself, facilitating the healing of others, pondering the lessons of spiritual leaders, communion with Nature, and life experiences.

As I see it, Spirit is our collective consciousness—our common guide. I use "Spirit," "God," and "the Divine" synonymously. Spirit pervades all; therefore, everything and everyone is beautiful and perfect, interconnected, and equally important. I am God; you are God. Within the overarching, collective Spirit, each human being is guided by his or her own, unique expression of Spirit. You have your own spirit, as do I. At every level, spirit is eternal and immutable.

Within each person's own spirit is the soul. Like the spirit, the soul is a timeless, immortal manifestation of the Divine, but in contrast to the spirit, the soul can change. The purpose of the soul is to learn and evolve as it travels a path guided by Spirit, and ultimately, to ascend. Your soul is the divine gift that allows you to make your unique and important contribution to the collective Spirit. Your soul is the life force that animates your physical body.

It is my soul, guided by Spirit, writing this chapter today. This book is among the infinite lessons that my soul will learn as I travel the course of countless lifetimes. When my evolution is complete, my soul will ascend into Spirit.

Your Journey

Your journey is not for spiritual growth; Spirit is fully grown. We are all on a path of self-discovery and *awakening* to

Spirit's design. The life you are living today is your vehicle for traveling that voyage. As your soul blossoms and unfolds—as you become what you are meant to be—you empower and enliven yourself and everyone else within the matrix.

We each have our own unique path, and nobody travels a smooth, straight and unobstructed road. What fun would that be? Every journey has peaks, valleys, bends and bumps. As we climb out of the valleys, we rarely get a straight shot to the top. On the way up we encounter dips and plateaus. As we descend into the deepest, darkest of valleys, we behold magnificent views on the way down. At the bottom we discover some of the most lush and unexpected beauty—beauty we could not see from the high points. Not until we reach the bottom can we find the treasures that the valley has to offer. Value your experience on the valley floor. If you only try to see the mountaintops, you will miss the gifts that are right within your reach.

The Buddha once said, "It is better to travel well than to arrive." The journey of the soul has no final destination. Follow your spiritual path as a lifelong journey of becoming, with less regard to getting.

We each have our own path to the Divine, and every path is valid. The way to reconnect with the Divine is to go inside. To quote the Dalai Lama: "There is no need for temples; no need for complicated philosophy. Our own brain, our own heart is our temple..."

We have made spirituality far too complicated and confusing. In Oby's life, spirituality was still simple. Nothing stood between Oby and Spirit. Oby saw Spirit in all things. When he gazed into the sky and watched the clouds float past on the way to their destination beyond the distant mountains, they touched his soul and enlivened his spirit. As he lay in the soft clover, basking in the warm sun, the experience of beholding such a heavenly parade stirred awe, wonder and love deep inside of him. He sensed that he, Fern, Scooter, the clouds, the clover, the mountains and all of Nature were equally important features in an endless landscape of possibility.

Oby never relied on any manuals, rituals or authority figures to understand God. It is a pretty safe bet that Fern never sat in full lotus on an imported designer meditation cushion, draped in a cashmere shawl, burning incense while meditating to new age music coming from her iPod. None of her friends ever genuflected in a church, lay prostrate before the Buddha, faced Mecca to pray, or bowed before the Wailing Wall. God spoke in clouds, sunsets, newborn babies...and rainbows. She still does.

If it feels right for you to follow a religion or spiritual tradition, then do so. Spiritual leaders are a gift to humanity. On my own journey, I have found deep inspiration in the teachings of The Dalai Lama, Martin Luther King Jr., Black Elk, Mahatma Gandhi, Mother Teresa, Thich Nhat Hanh and others. Many wonderful teachers can guide you along the path, but, ultimately, the path is yours. Nothing and no one stands between you and the Divine. You are the Divine.

Some people belong to meditation groups and some people go to a church, mosque, synagogue or temple every week. Groups, gurus, clergy and other teachers can help facilitate your process but, ultimately, your spiritual path is an internal one. If you go to a place of worship or practice with a meditation group, make sure it speaks to what is inside of you and helps to bring forth what your soul longs to express. No one can tell you what your soul should express. That is for you, alone, to discover.

An important part of my spiritual practice is the time I spend in Nature. To stand on a mountaintop in northern Idaho is to truly behold the Divine. I recall a day when I hiked to the top of a mountain called Mica Peak. The view from the summit was magnificent. I gazed at the majestic, snow-capped peaks of the Selkirk Mountains to the north, the Cabinet Mountains to the northeast and the Coeur d'Alenes and Bitterroots to the east. I could see the ski slopes on Schweitzer Mountain, Mount Spokane and Silver Mountain. Between my lofty lookout and the Selkirks stretched the tabletop-flat Rathdrum Prairie and, far to the south, the rolling contours of the Palouse country. There were sparkling lakes in every direction. The sky to the west was bright blue, and to the east, gray and foreboding. Towering thunderheads showered Mount Coeur d'Alene with a freezing spring rain. A stiff, frigid and enlivening north wind tore at my jacket, numbed my ears and threatened to steal my Seattle sombrero. As I sat against a rock eating my lunch, my dog, Sweetie, hunkered next to me to share my warmth, and poked her nose into the wind, enjoying the moment every bit as much as I. As I ate, I sized up the rugged Shasta Butte, a mile to the northwest, where Sweetie and I had been an hour earlier. The whole experience awed, humbled, and at the same time, exhilarated me. It was a deeply spiritual moment for me. I was alive! Connecting with Nature in all Her glory—hot and cold, in rain and sunshine, on towering peaks and in deep, dark canyons—brings me into communion with the wisdom that created me. When walking with Mother Nature, I am as able to touch the Divine as in my deepest meditations.

A Greater Power

The spiritual path is a path to a greater power, not a higher one. "Higher" power connotes a superior and separate entity; an ideal we cannot reach; a place we cannot go. We cannot even begin to comprehend the power that created the universe yet we all carry it within us. Within each of us is the artist that painted the aurora borealis and sculpted the Grand Canyon, and the genius that invented honeybees and solar systems. Human beings just like you and me gave us the great pyramids, space shuttles and post-it notes, as well as the civil rights movement and the Sunday comics.

We each represent an inextricable part of the Universal Intelligence that created us. So, how do we get in touch with it? First, remember this: the Divine is not Him, Her or IT; the Divine is you. Just go inside.

Meditation 101

Meditation puts you in touch with your divine inner self. There is no right or wrong way to meditate, nor is there a magic formula for meditating. You can go into a meditative state while sitting, lying down, standing, walking, or even running. Some people repeat a mantra; others hold a special stone in their hands; some gaze at a burning candle or visualize a placid pool of water. Many people do none of these. Meditation can take place in a serene natural setting, a quiet room with soft music, or amidst a hectic, noisy crowd.

When I was first learning to meditate, I was still in the Marines. One day I was on a bus full of raucous Marines as we were being transported from the ship that had just delivered us to Korea, to a base camp we would call home during a two-month training deployment. During the bus ride, I felt like practicing my meditation so I stuck my hands in my pockets, slouched down in my seat, pulled the bill of my camouflage cap down over my eyes and began to mentally repeat the mantra, "Om Namah Shivaya." Amid the surrounding cacophony, I soon found myself in a deep, blissful state of meditation. Everyone around me thought I was grabbing a quick catnap.

If you are just beginning to learn to meditate, explore different options and discover what works best for you. What I offer here are some simple, sensible thoughts on allowing meditation to happen, rather than a procedure or technique for "doing" it.

It helps to think of meditation as a deep state of physical relaxation, mental silence, inner awareness and complete presence with your soul. Meditation is a state of being, not an activity.

Many people use a mantra to help them reach a meditative state. One of the best-known and most commonly used mantras is the word, "Om," the primordial vibration of the Universe and the sound that pervades Nature. If chanting a mantra works for you, chant away. I generally do not use a mantra, but on those occasions when my intellectual mind keeps chattering away, I will use one. When I do, I usually repeat, "Just love...just love...just love..."

So...how to still the racing mind? I find it helps to let my thoughts roll through and regard them as background noise. We have all had the experience of immersing ourselves in a good book, oblivious to the sounds and activity happening all around us. The TV, other people's conversations, barking dogs—we may be aware of them, but we tune them out. Meditation can be the same way. As thoughts come to you, welcome and include them as part of your experience as you remain relaxed and focused within your meditative space. Thoughts can be bouncing around in the back of your mind and you will only be peripherally aware of them because you are in a deep state of meditation. Once you consciously start to approach meditation this way, you will be amazed at how well it works. Whatever technique you decide to use, be patient and try not to judge it by whether or not it works the first few times. It may take awhile so stick with it. If it feels right, it is right.

Just Meditate

Many times I have heard someone say, "I'll meditate on it." You can enjoy meditating without always having to meditate on a particular wish, subject or question. Just meditate. If you try to direct your meditation, you may limit it. When you meditate without an agenda, your innermost consciousness stays free to follow the wisdom of your soul. Years ago I always tried to focus my meditations. Every meditation had a sub-ject—an objective. I found that my thinking mind usually ended up going in a different direction from where I had planned, and my meditations were seldom very deep. The thoughts that came never seemed to be the thoughts I had planned. If I had a burning question or an important decision to make, I would meditate on it, but I rarely received a clear answer.

Once I simplified my meditation, I began to find greater joy in the journey and I am now able to go deeper than before. If I have a question, a concern, or a decision to make, occasionally meditation reveals an unequivocal answer; more often I gain a clear sense of my course of action, rather than a specific directive. Afterwards, my decision almost always turns out to have been the appropriate one.

One lesson I have learned the hard way is the futility of meditating with the specific intention to get rid of pain. An intense desire to get rid of pain brings a powerful pain consciousness into play. If you recall the lesson of the bike trail that I mentioned in the Introduction, you know that where you focus is exactly where you steer your life. Years ago when I was still in the Marines, I had a painful flare-up in my knee right before an upcoming physical fitness test. Marines never want to miss a PFT so I tried self-hypnosis to convince myself that I felt no pain. I repeated, "I feel no pain...I feel no pain..." As I was doing the three-mile run, I continued to repeat it. The pain got worse and worse, and I ended up not being able to finish the run. By concentrating so much on pain, I invited more pain into my life. In retrospect, I wonder what the outcome would have been if I had repeated, "I feel strong," or "I am super-man," or, "My feet have wings."

Starting a meditation practice can be like changing your diet. Anytime you change your routine it takes time to get in a groove. Then we experience ups and downs, ebbs and flows. For beginners, or for people who have tried meditating and "nothing happened," start with simple mindfulness of things that bring you joy and fulfillment. Whether an activity that you enjoy, spending time with a person or pet you love, or doing rewarding work, feel the joy and welcome the moment with love and gratitude. Your joy is an expression of your soul; an intimate connection with Spirit. Allow your spiritual practice to evolve as a natural extension of your joy.

Meditation Keeps You True to Yourself

Meditation is a key to success in life and health. Listening to the still voice within you unlocks your deepest potential and allows a wondrous journey to roll out before you. Personal success, however you choose to define it, is intricately interwoven with your spirit and your soul. In *The Success Principles*—one of the best personal growth books I have ever read—Jack Canfield says: "As you meditate, and become more spiritually attuned, you can better discern and recognize the sound of your higher self or the voice of God speaking to you through words, images, and sensations."

An enlivening, empowering spiritual practice allows you to grow and blossom in all areas of life. Staying committed to your spiritual practice will get you through the toughest of times and will help you stay true to your vision. A young chiropractor, freshly graduated from chiropractic college once called and asked me what advice I could offer to help her on her road to success. My advice consisted of one word, "meditate."

Starting a business comes with an array of challenges that can overwhelm even the most confident entrepreneur. Success is a process that takes time, effort, commitment and fortitude. Everybody starts with a starry-eyed vision of what they want to offer humanity and achieve for themselves. Then, as time drags on and obstacles arise, many people get tired and impatient, and lose sight of their vision. The principles they hold most dear are often those they let slide first. They get wrapped up in the daily difficulties that they perceive as reality, and lose sight of their own, *real* reality. So they compromise. They settle. As a result, any "success" they achieve is without true fulfillment. Why do you think burnout is such a huge issue in so many professions? People are not staying true to themselves. The famous motivational speaker and author, Zig Ziglar reminds us: "The chief cause of failure and unhappi-

ness is trading what you want most for what you want now."
Staying in touch with your soul's true calling will help you
attract what you want most in your life. The way to do that is
by listening to that clear, centered voice that speaks to you
from above down, inside out.

Finding the Time

Mahatma Gandhi is credited with saying, "I have so much
to do today, I need to meditate twice as long." And a famous
quote by Martin Luther conveys the same important message:
"I have so much to do today that I shall spend the first three
hours in prayer."

If you are a busy person, starting your day with meditation
or prayer will save you a lot of time in the long run. Twenty
minutes of quiet contemplation every day will pay you a huge
return in energy and clarity.

Spirit in Daily Life

Spirituality goes beyond meditation and prayer. The way
we live is even more important. A continuing, lifelong, self-
affirming approach to life brings happiness, health and success. A few years ago a young woman I know was despairing
that life never seemed to go her way. "If it's not one lousy
thing, it's another," she told me. I suggested that she adopt a
more positive internal dialogue. Her response was, "I tried
mantra-ing and it didn't work."

How far have we strayed when we look at a positive attitude as an intervention that does not work? A spiritual journey
is not as simple as repeating an affirmation a few times and—
poof—life is instantly hunky-dory. A positive outlook benefits
you best when it becomes your moment-to-moment way of

living rather than a procedure for getting. Think back to the story of our two friends, Win and Tank. Winifred chose to pursue success in the business world while her hapless friend, Tanicus, concentrated on avoiding failure. Although this gives Win a better chance for success, it remains possible that Win will tank and that Tank will win. Life sometimes plays out that way. But suppose we look at 1000 Wins and 1000 Tanks. Most Wins will succeed and some will fail. Many Tanks will succeed, but more Tanks, than Wins, will fail. Also consider how the Wins and Tanks each handle failure. The Tanks of the world are more likely to bemoan failure as their final outcome while the Wins recognize it as a valuable learning experience on their road to success. The Wins view life through a lens of optimism. Positive is how they live and, more importantly, it is who they are.

Mindfulness

Simple mindfulness can enhance this wondrous Earth journey of ours. Life has so much to offer and teach us. As you go through each day, carry with you a keen awareness and deep appreciation for each moment, person and experience. Let that sense of mindfulness and gratitude ease the pressures and complications of your daily life.

I once took a hike on one of my favorite lakeside trails on a spectacular Idaho summer day. The sky was clear and blue, a playful summer breeze teased the leaves on the trees, and Lake Coeur d'Alene was a clear and sparkling jewel. It was an afternoon to remember...for most people, anyway. As I paused to enjoy one of the many lovely views, a young man passed me, brow furrowed, talking on his cell phone. I smiled and waved but he paid me no heed. His important conversation made him oblivious to me, and the beauty and wonder surrounding him. He missed it all. A modern convenience had transformed him from a happy hiker into a stressed out, mindless pedestrian. His cell phone—or rather, his decision to take the call at that moment—robbed him of the joy, beauty, clarity and wisdom that Nature was offering him.

A friend of mine once told me a funny story with an important lesson about mindfulness. Quite some time ago, it seems, there was an old farmer who still had not had a telephone installed in his home. After many months of persuading, the farmer's son—now a grownup city slicker, wise to the ways of the world—finally convinced his cantankerous old father to get a telephone. "After all," the son had argued, "it's such a wonderful convenience." One day, the son paid a visit to the old homestead. After dinner, he and his father were sitting on the front porch enjoying the singing birds and watching the sun sink slowly beneath the rolling wheat fields. The phone rang. "Aren't you going to answer it?" asked the son. "Nope," replied the father. After seven rings the calling party hung up and the phone fell silent. "Why didn't you answer the phone?" asked the son. "Wasn't convenient," replied the wise old gentleman as he continued to enjoy the colorful sunset.

Gratitude

As you travel through life, carry with you an abiding sense of love and gratitude. As Dr. Emoto's water crystal experiments show, our consciousness is powerful enough to affect the physical state of matter—both positively and negatively. The water crystals offer us a vivid illustration of how powerful love and gratitude are. Dr. Emoto shares in his book that: "Indeed, there is nothing more important than love and gratitude in this world. Just by expressing love and gratitude, the water around us and in our bodies changes so beautifully. We want to apply this in our daily lives, don't we?"

Of course we do. Love is the real world; and we can feel grateful even when things are not going our way. Even major life challenges can be important steps along our spiritual path. When times get tough, it helps to keep in mind how important gratitude is and what a powerful force it is for unlocking your inherent potential.

Beautiful examples of the power of gratitude in the face of overwhelming challenges are the stories in the inspiring *Thank God I...* book series, In story after story, people describe, with deep gratitude, how cancer, rape, addictions, chronic disease, loss of loved ones, miscarriage and other experiences ultimately led to gifts in their lives that they would never have received otherwise. In the introduction to the first book, John Castagnini, the creator of the *Thank God I* series writes,

> *Beyond the pain, chaos and confusion of our circumstance exists true perfection. Thanking God is about finding this perfection. This place of thanking God might seem nearly impossible to find, but it is the only place we will find ourselves.*

Eating to Nourish Your Soul

The manner in which you receive, prepare, share and eat the foods that nourish you can add a beautiful dimension to your spiritual life. As the water crystals have shown us, the words we speak and the thoughts that run through our minds have a profound effect on the vibrational level of our food. If you welcome each meal and each bite with love and gratitude, the food will be a beautiful gift for your body. On the other hand, what will you be assimilating if you mindlessly shovel down a pizza while watching a shoot 'em up on TV? And how will a snack affect you if you eat it with a feeling of guilt for "cheating on your diet?"

We already know that love enhances the pleasure of eating. After all, the chocolate chip cookies that Grandma bakes with love are the most delicious cookies of all.

Your Mind, Heart and Soul Create Your Life

Life gives us what we feel and believe at a deep, core level. If you don't believe that we live in a universe of love and abundance, there is a process by which you can consciously change your beliefs. Start by putting into words what you want your new beliefs to be. The words must come from a place deep within you—a place of love, gratitude and trust. Then write, speak, visualize and feel your new beliefs throughout every aspect of your being—verbally, palpably, mentally and emotionally. Make a commitment to affirm your new beliefs every day, with the clear intention of allowing your life to roll out before you in the positive direction you have chosen.

Earlier, I related the story of an acquaintance who lamented, "I've tried mantra-ing and it didn't work." The reason it did not work was that her words were a superficial attempt at a quick fix. The universe doesn't work that way. We don't get to decide on all of the details in life. If we did, the world would be filled with a lot more billionaire supermodels involved in storybook romances.

The internal dialogue you carry throughout your day, every day, is more important than the "mantra-ing" you do for a couple of minutes in the morning until you decide that, "this stuff doesn't work."

The Buddha taught us:

The thought manifests as the word.
The word manifests as the deed.
The deed develops into habit.
And habit hardens into character.
So watch the thought and its ways with care,
and let it spring from love born out of concern for all beings.

Positive affirmations are an effective way to help manifest love, happiness, abundance and anything else you choose to include in your life's design. When you repeat your affirmations, it is not enough to merely regurgitate a string of words that you have memorized. Feel your intentions and behold their splendor in your mind's eye. Then act on them.

Affirmations are not an instant means to *get*. Your design grows from who and what you choose to be. In his visionary book, *Gesundheit!,* Patch Adams, M.D. points out, "Each of us chooses the background hues of his or her own portrait. A person can choose to be happy or miserable." Whether you are consciously aware of them or not, you repeat affirmations all day long. What you attract into your life is determined by the affirmations you choose. Your choice boils down to this: Will your affirmations be positive and empowering, or gloomy and foreboding? We all have an endless inner dialogue programming our human software. If you constantly think: "Oh woe is me. If it's not one thing, it's another," so shall your life unfold. Optimistic thoughts work the same way. Make a commitment to reveal life's unlimited love, peace and success, and those treasures will be your reward.

Love and abundance are the reality of the world. Repeating positive affirmations reconnects you with your very essence, and will bring forth the love, peace, vibrance and joy that reside there every moment of your life.

It will help if your affirmations are of your own design. Many self help books contain some excellent affirmations that can be good starting points. Use those that feel right for you, and then let your own affirmations evolve from them. You will manifest exactly what you affirm, so your choice of words is important. Avoid phrases that begin with, "I will...," "I want...," or "I need." They can create a perpetual state of waiting, want and need. State your affirmations in the present tense, as an acknowledgement that what you envision already exists within the matrix. Words such as, "I have...," and "I am...," will realize your vision.

When I discuss the need to phrase affirmations in the present tense, as a statement of truth, people sometimes protest and tell me, *"I can't say that I am already enjoying vibrant health and financial abundance. That would be a lie. Doc, you know I can barely stand up straight...and I never know from one month to the next whether I'll be able to pay my rent."*

Understand that affirmations are not meant to be an accurate statement of your current circumstances. In designing an affirmation, you have already decided that your present day situation is not the reality you desire. Your affirmations are statements to *affirm* the truth that you have decided to create for yourself. Your affirmations are an expression of your truest truth.

With all of that in mind, I will share a few of my own affirmations:

- *"I enjoy a constant state of robust health, physical strength, vitality, well-being, strong, clear vision, and boundless energy."*
- *"I live my life on a solid foundation of love, gratitude and trust. I grow, thrive, serve and prosper from that same foundation."*
- *"Today and every day I am mindful of every moment and present with every person."*
- *"My deepest intention with all people is to love, to serve and to empower."*
- *"I am loved because I am love. I am love because I am loved."*
- *"I am blessed with enduring faith, hope, love, life, light, joy, happiness, peace, tranquility, grace, serenity, gratitude, inner strength, courage, humility, mindfulness, wisdom and trust."*

The last affirmation has evolved over a number of years. It started eight years before I began writing this book with, *"Faith, hope, love, life, light."* Over time, I added others, one or two at a time, as life's insights presented them to me. Who knows how much farther it may go? That is what I mean when I say to allow your own affirmations to come forth.

Just Love Yourself

One of the most important early steps in deep, core healing is to learn to *just* love yourself. Love everything about yourself—your body, your appearance, your gifts, your challenges—everything. Remember, at your core, you are love. Just love.

Engaging in a moment-to-moment, lifelong process of bringing this core essence to light is a beautiful, powerful, empowering path for healing.

Just love yourself as a being of beauty and perfection. Note that I have not said to "accept" yourself. Just love yourself without feeling obligated to accept or reject anything. I also did not tell you to love yourself "just the way you are." Just love yourself without regard to what you are, what you were, what you hope someday to be, or what your fears tell you that you may someday become. We can love ourselves today, in this moment, and still work to grow and evolve in our lives. To quote Ralph Waldo Emerson: "These roses beneath my window make no reference to former roses or better ones. They are for what they are. They exist with God today."

Exist with God today—just love yourself.

Oby's Wisdom

- You are a uniquely beautiful and perfect expression of the Divine.

- Your spiritual journey is to a greater power within you, not a higher one beyond you.

- The Divine is not Him, Her or It. You are the Divine.

- Meditation puts you in touch with your divine inner self.

- Rather than meditating on your concerns, just meditate.

- Be mindful of every moment, every person and every experience.

- Welcome each meal and each bite with love and gratitude.

- Your words are your life.

- Just love yourself.

Chapter Seven

Mother Nature
Packed Us a Lunch

> *Food is an important part of a balanced diet.*
> Fran Lebowitz

Oby and Fern had a height and weight chart hanging on the wall above their bathroom scale.

Just kidding.

Oby and Fern innately knew what many of us have lost sight of. We eat to turn our health inside out. Glaringly obvious, yes, but we seem to have forgotten.

For many, food is a battle. Almost all of us have been on a diet at some point in time. Some people always seem to be on a diet—and usually not a consistent one. Opinions as to what comprises healthy nutrition change from time to time, and our eating habits usually follow the latest theory or fad. How many people have stayed on their 1970's low cal diet through the low fat and low carb eras?

This chapter offers you a simple solution: Never go on a diet again. When I say, "don't go on a diet," I am referring to the intention, not to the behavior. Almost anybody can benefit from healthier eating habits. The important thing is the intention—to incorporate better nutrition into your life for the health benefits, and not to fight yourself.

Excess weight is just another example of IT. So many diet plans, diet books and weight loss programs exist that it would probably be impossible to count them all. Low cal, low fat, low carb, slow carb, raw food, beer and cookies—the list continues to expand.

And they all work.

But none of them work.

That is, they all work if you stick to them, but virtually no one sticks to them over a lifetime. I'm not joking about the beer and cookies diet. When I was a student at the University of Idaho, my good friend, Bill, was famous for his beer and cookies diet. He wanted to maintain a healthy weight, but he knew that beer and cookies, on top of everything else he ate and drank, would probably cause him to gain weight. He decided to do away with the unnecessary foods and just stick with the beer and cookies (augmented with an occasional bowl of yogurt). He stuck with it religiously for a good two months. Many of the caring young women he knew provided him with support in the way of home-baked oatmeal raisin cookies. In a pinch, between batches of homemade cookies, he managed to get by with store-bought vanilla wafers. Whichever cookies he had on his plate, he washed them down with his favorite beer, "whatever's cheap and cold." I would never suggest a strict regimen of beer and cookies as a healthy approach to maintaining your ideal weight, and I doubt the beer and cookies diet ever graced the pages of a peer-reviewed nutritional journal. If it had, I would have enjoyed reading the letters to the editor in the following issue. Bill never tried to pass his diet off as serious; it was just a fun college guy thing. But Bill did follow his diet for two months, and he did meet his objective. It supports the point I am trying to get across. In terms of weight management, lots of diet plans will work, no matter how kooky or unhealthy. The challenge is sticking to a regimen...for the rest of your life.

A number of years ago I read a sobering statistic: Losing weight and keeping it off permanently is more difficult than overcoming cancer. Is that a wakeup call, or what? I am not here to roll a dark cloud of discouragement into anyone's life. For many who have struggled with weight issues for years or even decades, that dark cloud is already there. I provide that statistic to illustrate how important it is for us to change our mindset.

I enjoy presenting wellness lectures to organizations in my community. When I get to the part of my lecture where I discuss nutrition, I ask, "How many of you have ever gone on a diet?" Regardless of the audience, almost all adults raise their hands. I follow with: "Now, how many of you enjoy going on a diet? I don't mean the end result of having lost weight, but the process of dieting itself—how many of you enjoy that?" Rarely has a hand ever risen.

What is the most common reason that people go on diets? The dreaded mirror. What do we do when we look in the mirror every morning? We take inventory of everything that we judge to be wrong with ourselves. We scrutinize our grey hairs hoping that no new ones have sprouted since the last inventory. We tug on wrinkles to try to smooth them out—only to have them spring back—and we pinch our midsections and thighs to check out how much of IT is there.

Often our observations are accompanied by a self-destructive judgment such as:

"Geez, you look like #*¢π!"
"Morning, Porky."

Eventually we proclaim for the first, tenth or hundredth time: "That's it. No more. I'm gonna lose this weight once and for all. Time to go on a diet." Sometimes the decision to go on a diet is not because of a weight issue. It can be a therapeutic diet for trying to overcome a disease of some sort. Even then, the focus is on the disease. We want to make IT go away. It boils down to the same thing. People usually go on diets because they do not like themselves.

Often a new diet begins with yet another book, article, glossy magazine ad, clinically proven product, or quick and easy program that promises to help you lose IT, and keep IT off forever. Then the process proceeds as it has so many times before.

Excitement.

Self discipline.

Starting to lose IT (weight).

Lookin' pretty good.

Starting to lose it (excitement and self discipline).

Gaining IT back.

Resignation.

Guilt and self-loathing.

Again.

Why Diets Fail

Dr. Mark's definition of "dieting:"

The process of doing something you don't like...to take care of something you don't like.

What are the odds of that succeeding?

It will be much more self-affirming for you to remember The Basic Truth: You are beautiful and perfect. As I said earlier, this is not meant to be a magical incantation that will lead you to an instant fix. What I am offering is a new, more positive, more empowering way of thinking. Embrace yourself as a beautiful and perfect being, and live your life from that perspective. Then imagine what your life and health will be like in 5...10...25...50 years from now, compared to what it will be like if you keep loathing yourself. Just love yourself and do everything you do—including eating—from that place of self-love.

The narrow focus on weight loss alone can be very unhealthy. When we only worry about losing IT, we are mainly concerned about appearance, not health. We are endlessly inundated with images of svelte, tanned, smiling, supermodels, male and female, gracing advertisements for everything from bikinis to junk food. We expect that we should look that way, too. This ideal comes from a skewed perspective of what perfection is supposed to look like. Many models have unhealthy diets and lifestyles just to maintain their look. Much of what we see is artificial. It is no secret that many magazine photo spreads are airbrushed and digitally enhanced.

The supermodels, male and female, that we see on magazine covers are professionals. Their livelihood and reputation depend on their maintaining their physical appearance. Many of us expect ourselves to look like the pros. That is true even when we have no such expectations in other parts of our lives.

I love bicycling but I know Lance Armstrong will never eat my dust on a tough climb in the Alps. As a matter of fact, were I ever to find myself ascending L'Alp D'Huez with Lance, he would pull away so fast I would never have the pleasure of eating *his* dust. I am not a professional bike racer so it would be ridiculous for me to try to be the cyclist that Lance is. I am not a professional body builder, either. Why then, should I expect to have the same physique as the cover model on a fitness magazine?

The Gunny

People sometimes sacrifice their health when they only worry about losing IT. When I was a captain in the Marines, we had a Gunnery Sergeant in my outfit who did not meet the official Marine Corps height and weight standards. Back then, the Marines had a program known as the Weight Control Program. Despite its official wording it played out as appearance-oriented, and had little to do with health and performance.

Even though the Gunny was deemed overweight, he was in pretty decent shape. He easily passed his semiannual physical fitness tests and he could perform all of the duties the Marine Corps required of him. That didn't matter when the Gunny hopped on the scale. Time after time, the doc had to slide the weight farther along the bar than was allowed. There was no avoiding it; we had to put the Gunny on weight control. Once on weight control, a Marine was given a certain amount of time to lose a specified amount of weight. Failure to lose the weight meant a discharge from the Marine Corps. Despite a great deal of counseling, cajoling, joining the Run for Lunch Bunch, and weekly weigh-ins, the Gunny went quite a long period of time without losing any weight. He eventually found himself with one month left and still a long way to go to meet the standard. He was facing the end of an honorable and productive career because of that stubborn spare tire. Out of desperation, he went on a crash diet. He lost a lot of weight in that last month and met his objective.

He succeeded!
He lost IT!
He was off weight control!
Hooray for the Gunny!
Hooray for the Weight Control Program!

Then, the Gunny failed his next physical fitness test. He looked better in his uniform, but he had weakened himself so much in his desperation weight loss that he could no longer accomplish his mission. We had a good-looking, physically unfit leader of Marines. My purpose for telling this story is not to criticize the Marine Corps. I love the Marines. They have my deepest respect and admiration, and always will. Physical fitness is paramount in the Marines, and I would never suggest that Marines be allowed to have unhealthy bodies. I tell the Gunny's story to show that the ultimate purpose of the old weight control program—although ostensibly to improve health—was really to make Marines look better. What happened with the Gunny did not serve the Marine Corps and it certainly did not serve the Gunny. Thankfully, the Marine Corps has a better program today than the one we had back then.

The Gunny's story is a reflection of our society. Many people resort to unhealthy, even dangerous lifestyles in their quest for that ever-elusive Hollywood physique. People have even died on that quest. The obsession with losing IT sometimes turns *off* life.

Good looks, as defined by fashion and fitness magazines, are mere judgments. When you eat for the vitality that fresh, whole foods give you, rather than dieting for looks, your health and life will improve. Our bodies are not just for display. They are where we live, work and play.

Look Beyond the Numbers

Even though height and weight charts have been designed by health professionals, they provide an uncertain, incomplete framework for assessing health. Plenty of "overweight" people are actually quite healthy. And many thin people, who are not technically underweight, have compromised their health because of what they do to maintain their "healthy" weight. A study published in the Journal of the American Medical Association (JAMA) in April 2005, stated that "modestly overweight" people have a "lower risk of death" than people whose weight falls within normal weight limits on a chart. But hold on. This isn't a green light for you to speed down to the nearest ice cream parlor for a super double hot fudge sundae. I mention the study only to emphasize that guidelines are far from exact. The results of the JAMA study suggest that maybe the experts who drew up the chart may not have gotten it quite right. Such charts and guidelines are never more than a best guess so why be tied to them? Do you even need your scale and your chart? They serve only as tools to quantify IT.

Now, about your mirror. Of course you can use it to make sure you are impeccably groomed and neatly clothed, but stop taking inventory of your perceived flaws. Use your mirror to love and admire yourself. Every morning before I leave for my office I check the mirror to make sure my hair looks neat. I slick down my ever-present cowlick and head for the door. Then when I get to my office and take off my hat and coat, I recheck myself before people start coming in the door. I admire my cowlick, slick it down again and prepare to spend the day turning health inside out.

Order from Nature's Menu

Now we come to the question, "How should I eat?" An endless and bewildering stream of new diet programs keeps us bouncing from one quick and easy plan to the next. Today's new plan often contradicts yesterday's. Theories abound. Debates rage. In any of the debates, both sides can roll out reams of scientific research, case studies and compelling testimonials to defend their position.

Should I be a vegetarian, or even a vegan, or is meat OK?

Do I have to go raw or is it safe to have a hardboiled egg with my breakfast?

Low fat, low carb, low cal, or...what?

Who has the answer? *Nature.* When Mother Nature put us on this planet, she packed us a lunch. Nutrition was pretty simple back in Oby's day. Oby ate what Nature provided. He never had the need to scrutinize complex lists of unpronounceable ingredients or analyze any confusing nutritional information. All foods were organic, in season and locally produced.

Our Paleolithic predecessors remind us of a simple and important lesson: Eat fresh, whole, natural foods.

The Most Important Nutrient

The single most important nutrient—and the one most lacking in our diet of processed and packaged foods is *life*. Processing robs food of its life essence and often adds unnecessary synthetic ingredients. That can be true with junk food as well as many "health" foods.

Almost anyone reading this book knows that organic foods are superior to nonorganic ones. Organic foods are free of the toxic fertilizers, pesticides, hormones and other chemicals that non-organic foods contain. More importantly, organic foods do not rely on artificial means to become delicious and healthful. They grow and develop by maximizing their own life potential, and by expressing their own beauty and perfection. Organic foods are more alive.

Another important lesson we can learn from Oby and Fern is to enjoy fruits and vegetables that are in season and locally grown. The foods that Mother Nature has to offer right now in your own area are in resonance with you—they are tuned to the same frequency. The well-known Doctor of Oriental Medicine and author, Dr. Michael Tierra once wrote of an experience he had that illustrates this point perfectly. He was on a trip from the Bay Area to Southern California and had a bag of fresh, juicy oranges to enjoy on his drive. As his journey progressed and he got further and further away from home, the oranges he was eating began to cause him to develop cold symptoms. His body was dialing in to a new energy field, but the oranges, having already been harvested, remained stuck on their old frequency.

The fruits and vegetables that you bought from your local farmer's market this morning are playing clear and beautiful music. In contrast, the produce that was harvested and frozen months ago half way across the continent, is coming in fuzzy and broken.

Genetically Modified—Just Another Processed Food

The subject of genetically modified foods brings up another contentious debate where scientific studies are at odds. Who do we believe? Consider this: We know that Nature constantly evolves. Our food supply—both animal and vegetable—has evolved right along with us. Genetically modified foods have taken a different road. In a way, they are yet another example of a processed food. Just because they poke up out of the soil somewhere does not automatically make them natural. Even some of the ingredients in Twinkies had their start in a fertile field at some point in time.

Supplements

There are differing schools of thought on the necessity for taking supplements. They have their place but I feel that people depend on them way too much. Personally, I virtually never use vitamin supplements or commercially produced herbal remedies. I do enjoy preparing meals with various fresh herbs. Decide what is right for you with the understanding that, although some are better than others, supplements are processed products. Never delude yourself into believing that pills and capsules will adequately compensate for poor nutrition. We call them "supplements" because they supplement healthy foods. The bottom line: Eat a balance of fresh, whole, natural foods.

I realize that eating exclusively like I have described may be a challenge for many people—at least at first. So just do your best. If you haven't visited the organic section of your favorite supermarket recently, check it out the next time you are there. Organics are becoming more available and more affordable as their popularity increases. A pound of organic broccoli, a bunch of organic spinach or whatever fresh, organic produce happens to be on sale this week might very well be cheaper than that bag of store brand tater tots in in your cart.

If you believe that you can save money by buying cheaper processed foods, think again. Sure, you may pay less at the check stand today, but the harmful health effects you experience down the road will make "cheap" junk food the most expensive food you will ever buy.

To change eating habits you have had for a long time, take it one small, pleasurable step at a time. Pick up some of the delicious, healthy foods you want to add to your diet and stop worrying so much about what to give up. Adding value to your life is much more empowering than deprivation. On your next trip to the grocery store, spend a little extra time in the produce section. Find foods there that you like. Take some of them home...and enjoy.

One final thought: lighten up! Avoid the stress of rigidity and austerity by allowing yourself a treat from time to time. Because I just love myself, every now and then I like to treat myself to a couple of scoops of cool, sweet, smooth moose tracks ice cream. Delicious! And because I just love myself, I only do that every now and then.

Adopt your healthier way of eating as a lifelong commit-ment—a lifestyle rather than a program. As with any process, there will be ebbs and flows. Flow with the process, stay committed and let it progress.

Oby's Wisdom

- Let self-love guide your eating choices.

- Your body is not just for display; it's where you live, work and play.

- The most important nutrient is life.

- Choose organic, locally grown foods first.

- "Cheap" junk food is the most expensive food you will ever buy.

- Adding value is more enjoyable and more effective than deprivation.

- Allow yourself an occasional treat.

- Honor the ebbs and flows of the process, and stay committed.

Chapter Eight

Fun, Fitness and Life

> *I am convinced that life in a physical body is meant to be an ecstatic experience.*
> **Shakti Gawain**

What do you love to do—which physical activities give you the greatest pleasure? Go out and enjoy them! There you have it—your perfect exercise program, custom tailored to fit your unique needs.

If you have ever read books or articles about exercising, you have probably run across something like this: "To benefit from an exercise routine, you must exercise at 65% to 85% of your target heart rate for at least 20 minutes, three times a week. To calculate your target heart rate you must first determine your maximum heart rate, which is derived by..."

All of that may true and valid, and I tip my hat to those who spent the time and effort to figure it out, along with the many scientific guidelines for weight training, aerobic activity and other forms of exercise. This information is great for anyone interested in using it. I sometimes use a heart rate monitor when I run or bike. Other people have no interest in calculating their target heart rate, and are even less inclined to spend their money on a heart rate monitor to keep track of it. No one should expect them to.

The Gym and the Trout Stream

It would probably take more than ten fingers to count all of your friends, acquaintances and relatives that have plunged into a workout regimen but quit after a short time because they lacked the motivation. In too many lives, exercise without joy has become yet another stress. Take Bob, for example. Bob is a pretty healthy guy but a couple of months ago he realized he had not been active in quite some time. He was starting to feel the effects of too much sitting around. His belt had gotten a little bit tighter and he had a lot less energy than before. Bob decided it was time to make some healthy changes in his life. One day, on the way home from work, he swung by the local fitness center and signed up. They had a special deal for new members that week.

Brock, one of the fitness trainers, showed him around. They had lots of shiny high tech resistance machines, row after row of state-of-the-art computerized cardio equipment, a huge room full of free weights, and big TV sets tuned to news and sports. Bob was excited knowing he could stay up to date on the stock market or watch the playoffs while the treadmill kept track of his heart rate and how many calories he was burning. After Brock bid him farewell, Bob browsed through their pro shop and bought some stylish new workout attire. He also picked up an impressive training log. He eyed the heart rate monitors for a few minutes but decided not to buy one because the cardio machines had them built in. He walked happily to his car humming *"Let's Get Physical* ..." As soon as he hit the freeway, he polished off a couple of the energy bars he had grabbed at the checkout stand and washed them down with a bottle of a bright blue energy drink. He was not sure what flavor it was supposed to be but it tasted good and it sure looked cool. Bob was motivated and eager to start working out at that sparkling facility...next week...as soon as he tied up those loose ends on the Watkins account.

There was only one problem. Bob has never enjoyed working out in gyms. He has belonged to them before, but he never stuck with it. In the end, the only thing that any of his gym memberships ever developed in him was guilt. And once again, Bob's pattern continued...

The following Monday morning arrived with Bob's clock radio waking him up an hour and a half earlier than usual. He bounded out of bed, hurried through his morning routine and skipped out the door, anxious to get to the gym. He had a great workout. When his alarm went off on Wednesday, he hit the snooze button. Then he hit it again ten minutes later. A half an hour after that, he finally rolled out of bed, deciding he would not read the newspaper that morning. That would make up for most of the time he lost to the snooze button. After all, Bob reasoned, pretty soon he would be watching news on the gym's big screen TV anyway. He made it to the fitness center almost as early as planned and he had a pretty decent workout. Then on Friday, Bob could not drag himself out of bed early enough to make it to the gym. Skipping his workout made him feel a little bit guilty, but he rationalized it by remembering what a tough week it had been. He made it to the gym the following Monday, but it was getting tougher and tougher every day. On

Wednesday, Bob's glassy eyes completely missed the beautiful sunrise as he drove to the gym. When his alarm sounded off that morning, it was only by sheer force of will that he was able to drag himself out of bed after a couple of snoozers. Bob was stressed. He disliked getting up that early and he was not having much fun at the gym. He felt guilty blowing it off because he had spent all that money on his membership. Plus, he had that great training log—it would be a shame to let that go to waste. Besides, what would Brock think?

Bob wished he could be like his new friend, Todd. Todd always goes big and works up a serious sweat. Every day! And as he walks cheerfully out the door—right after making a stop at the juice bar for his Super Power Mojo, with extra dashes of bee pollen and whey protein—he always has a spring in his step and bright smile on his face. "Why can't I be that motivated?" Bob wonders.

Here's why, Bob. Todd loves the gym. You don't.

What does Bob love to do? Fish! Plus, his girlfriend, Terry, just bought a shiny new Electra beach cruiser. Bob thinks it would be fun to get one too, so they can spend time together, pedaling some of the scenic local bike trails. Another sport Bob has always enjoyed is bowling. If Bob spent time doing what he enjoyed, he would hardly ever have to struggle to get out of bed in the morning. But he thinks they are not exercise—not really. At least, not according to Brock.

True, maybe they are not as intense as sweating in air-conditioned comfort for 30 minutes at level ten on the computerized exercise bike, but they are physical exercise. Fishing, biking and bowling are a lot more beneficial than playing dodge the gym. Bowling every Tuesday, taking two or three leisurely bike rides a week and pulling on the ol' waders on the weekend will be better for Bob than working out at the gym for a couple of weeks and then laying off for another six or eight months.

The First Rule of Fitness: "Play First!"

I have a good friend named Chic (never call him Charles) who is the most hardcore outdoor enthusiast I have ever known. Hiking, mountain biking, kayaking, skiing, you name it; Chic excels. He is about sixty-ish and is a most impressive physical specimen. What I love the most about Chic is his motto, "play forever, work whenever." To him, life is about fun, not toil. Don't get me wrong, Chic works hard at his job (although he would vehemently deny it). He is an icon at Camera Corral, the premier camera shop in Coeur d'Alene, Idaho. Local photography buffs know that if you ever have a question about cameras or photography, Chic is the guy to ask.

Chic often leads organized hikes for a club called The Spokane Mountaineers. Only the hardiest of the hardy dare to venture into the wilderness with Chic. He likes to spend as much time as possible off of the beaten path. Chic has taken the concept of bushwhacking to a whole new level. Those who have trekked with him have dubbed it "Chic-whacking." A few years ago, Chic led a small but enthusiastic band of us on a merry little jaunt in the rugged and breathtaking Selkirk Mountains in the panhandle of Idaho. The hike lasted about 12 hours, with ten of those hours off trail. For most of the day, the rest of us were groaning and sweating, but Chic's smile never faded. The point is that, although Chic engages in more rigorous physical activity than almost anyone, he never follows anything you would call an exercise "program" or "regimen." He just plays. And he is probably in better shape than 99% of

Americans. I once asked Chic how he finds the time to devote to all of the outdoor activities he enjoys. With a beaming smile and a twinkle in his eye he offered a snippet of simple wisdom so brilliant that I have adopted it as my First Rule of Fitness: *"Play first!"*

"Whoever Can Hurt the Most, Wins."

By no means am I suggesting that no one ever follow a structured training program. If you have one you enjoy, keep at it. I have a friend named Ethan who is a professional mountain bike racer as well as an accomplished competitor in road racing, time trial, criterion and cyclocross. He owns seven bicycles of different types, and he rides all of them...a lot. In an average year Ethan will log about 9,000 to 10,000 miles in the saddle.

Needless to say, as a pro, Ethan follows a rigorous and scientific training program. He always uses a heart rate monitor to guide his training intensity. The wheel of Ethan's road bike is equipped with a sophisticated computerized hub that measures wheel speed and torque, and computes the power—measured in watts—that Ethan pumps out as he rides. Riders of his caliber can generate more power than some radio stations. The hub transmits the information to a small digital data display on the handlebars for Ethan to monitor as he rides. After each ride, he downloads the data onto a computer and creates a profile of the ride that he can analyze to fine tune his training.

The volume and intensity of Ethan's training is just as impressive as the technology. His fit and athletic wife, Shannon, loves his rest days because she can actually ride with him. (A rest day for Ethan might mean that he only goes out for a one or two hour "easy spin.") Shannon is a marathoner, an Ironman triathlon finisher, and a strong cyclist in her own right, but an easy spin for Ethan is a workout for Shannon.

Ethan's team has a saying they follow on race day to motivate themselves to excel: "Whoever can hurt the most, wins."

In other words, whoever can dig the deepest and push the hardest brings home the gold.

Be Like Ethan

Ethan has another saying, "I do what I love and I love what I do." To enjoy a peak level of fitness, health and well-being, you do not need to follow a training regimen as strict and challenging as Ethan's (but you can if you want to), and you will never need to out-hurt anyone. The example to follow is this: Do what you love and love what you do.

Get Moving!

Multiple choice question: The most important benefit of exercise is

1. Strength
2. Endurance
3. Flexibility
4. None of the above

Answer: 4. None of the above

The most important aspect of exercise is motion. While strength, endurance and flexibility are key ingredients of overall fitness, and wonderful benefits of physical activity, the best part of exercise is that it gets us moving. Nature designed us to be dynamic. We are at our best at the high vibratory state brought about by motion. Today, our challenge is that most of us spend the day on the couch, in the car and in front of a computer, rather than hunting and gathering from dawn to dusk. Our sedentary lifestyle is at odds with our dynamic nature. The human body thrives on motion. Spending an afternoon planting flowers or taking a leisurely walk through the neighborhood park are both wonderful forms of exercise. Motion is life.

Body, Mind, Emotions, Spirit—One Synergistic Whole

Physical activity is important for the whole person, not just for the physical body. Our spiritual, mental, emotional and physical aspects are intricately intertwined. Your mind, emotions and spirit dwell in your physical body. The better each one works, the better they all work; when you exercise your body, you also sharpen your mind and nurture your soul. Physical activity makes us feel good deep inside. Many of the profound pearls I proffer on these pages have sprung forth as I was spinning, striding, stretching or splitting firewood. In fact, the clever sentence you just read came to me while I was taking a break from the computer screen and enjoying one of my favorite yoga exercises, the seven motions of the spine.

Physical activity enables you to venture into layers of your psyche that would otherwise be out of reach. Why? Because being active is part of your core essence. We are designed to move. We must move. All living bodies are enlivened by physical activity. That goes for all of us—including you. The greatest benefit of exercise is that it elevates your spirit, not just your heart rate.

Effort

Building a vibrant life calls for commitment and self-discipline. By its very nature, exercise requires that you exert yourself. But this does not mean that exercise has to be a chore. Just play! Playing makes your effort fun. Have you ever watched children on a playground? They are working hard while having a great time. None of us has ever heard a child say: "No thanks, Dad. I don't feel like going to the playground today...too much work." When I run or hike up a scenic mountain trail it takes a lot of hard work. I love every second of it because a backcountry trail is one of my favorite places to play.

It takes effort for busy people to set aside time for physical activity. One of the dilemmas we face in our hectic world is that activities like exercise and meditation—the ingredients in life that are so critical to allow us to stay healthy amid all of the stress—are the very things we let slide when we start feeling a time crunch. As a result, we sacrifice the things we need the most, right when we most need them.

If your chosen physical activity is not one you enjoy, it will be all too easy to put it on the back burner and leave it there. Why would anyone take time away from something they need to do so they can go do something they don't want to do? If you are getting off of work at 6:30 in the evening and you still planned to get in two hours on the bike for your triathlon training, I hope triathlon is a pursuit that you love.

Harvesting the Couch Potato

What about people who are not physically inclined? That can be a tough one because of the inertia that builds as couch time increases. Remember what I said earlier—the need and want to be active is part of our core essence. Getting a couch potato to become physically active requires no more than a reconnection with one's true nature.

Oby, Fern, Scooter and their friends were all active. They had to be. If they had slept late every morning then lounged around all day, they never would have survived. Their lives depended on staying active. So does yours.

The couch potato is a relatively recent phenomenon. Couches have been around for about 4000 years, whereas couch potatoes did not exist in significant numbers until the 20th century. For you sedentary souls out there who want to get moving, try this process:

Step 1: *Pick up remote; hit "off" button.*
Step 2: *Go out and play.*

Think back to when you enjoyed being physically active, and remember how much fun you had. If you enjoyed it then, you still do. Recapture that joy. Even if you have never enjoyed physical activity, that desire is somewhere inside of you. Your challenge is to reveal it. If you are in poor shape, take it slow. Perhaps you look back with pride to the days when your opponents feared your high flying spikes on the base paths. Be careful, though. If those days were 20 years and 100 pounds ago, don't plan on making any hard slides into home plate by next week. Start by playing catch and batting tennis balls against the side of your garage, and then allow the process to progress naturally.

"But at the end of the day, I just wanna relax."

This is a lament I have heard on occasion. I can understand the sentiment, but lethargy is not equivalent to relaxation.

When I go out for a run or a hike, one of the most important reasons is that it helps me escape the pressures of the day. After a great run and a long stretch, I enjoy a state of relaxation that surfing the net will never provide. Fun exercise—within your capabilities—is more relaxing than sitting around. Among the many benefits of regular exercise are reduction of stress, improved mental focus, increased energy levels and improved quality of sleep. A long evening of channel surfing agitates you and drains your energy. A couple of my favorite reasons for running are that it clears my mind and mellows me out.

This does not mean that your waking hours need to be a ceaseless flurry of activity. Exercise must be balanced with adequate rest. The act of running, itself, illustrates how to find equilibrium between rest and exercise. In *ChiRunning*, one of the most bookmarked and highlighted books that I own, author Danny Dreyer teaches a running technique that decreases the effort required for running. As he points out, "It doesn't mean that there's *no* effort, just no *unnecessary* effort."

"I Love Hills!"

In the late 1980's, I lived on the island of Okinawa and I had a bicycling buddy named Mike. We rode together often and both shared the same aversion to hills. Now, you must understand that cyclists find it pretty hard to avoid hills on Okinawa. Okinawa is basically a mountain range sticking up out of the Pacific Ocean, so steep hills are part of the deal there. One Saturday morning, before one of our long weekend rides, I was reading an article in *Bicycling* magazine that listed various training tips for climbing hills. One of the paragraphs was entitled, "I love hills." The paragraph recommended always telling yourself that you love hills, especially when you are approaching a tough climb. When I met Mike that morning for our ride, it turned out that he had just read the same article. So we tried it. On that first morning we groaned our way up the grueling climbs as we always had (it wasn't—poof—magic), but over the course of several months we grew to genuinely love them. Instead of plodding up them with a resigned whimper, we attacked even the steepest hills with relish. As we progressed, we became a couple of first class mountain goats.

If you never feel like getting physical, come up with an affirmation. Try something like: "I love my afternoon walks," or "I always enjoy my morning yoga practice," or "I can't wait to shoot hoops after work." Make the affirmation about an activity that you enjoy, or at least used to enjoy, and repeat it every day. By getting back in touch with what gives you joy, you will encourage your true, physically active self to emerge.

Listen To Your Body

True or false: "Before starting this or any other exercise program, always consult your physician." Answer: False.

I am often asked questions like, "Is it OK for me to be doing this?" or "Should I be doing that?" My answer almost always includes this guidance: "Listen to your body." As a doctor, I will almost never recommend that someone quit doing something they love, because that would impose a significant stress into their life. In those cases where people may be served by modifications to their physical activities, I help them tune into their Innate Wisdom that knows, better than I, what is safe and unsafe for them.

Fern never strapped a heart rate monitor to her wrist, but whenever she hurried back to the cave with a heavy bag of acorns slung over her shoulder, she knew when to slow down and when she could speed back up. She also knew when to switch shoulders.

Listening to your body goes deeper than whether or not you feel discomfort. Your body may tell you in a voice other than pain that an injury is sneaking up on you. Tennis elbow and shin splints show up well after athletes' bodies have started telling them that the injury is approaching. Conversely, some forms of exercise can benefit us even when they feel uncomfortable or painful when we do them properly. Stretching and weight lifting are two examples. We have all heard the term, "It hurts so good." Before I go on, please understand that I am not espousing the "no pain, no gain" philosophy. I am saying that pain is neither good nor bad all by itself. Pain is a message, but not your body's only voice.

Physicians can be a great source of advice when you decide that seeking such advice is right for you. If you feel the need to ask, then by all means ask. In addition to doctors, there are other great sources of information and advice. If I have a concern with a certain yoga posture, I ask my well trained and experienced yoga teacher, not a doctor. As far as I know, yoga is not part of the curriculum in most western medical schools.

Ultimately, your greatest source of wisdom is your own Innate Intelligence. Unfortunately, most people have lost the ability to listen to their bodies because we're so often told to consult a physician before we do anything.

Your body's cues can be so subtle—*whispers*—that you may miss them if you are not paying attention. Sadly, most people have become clueless as to how to tune in to them. When I first tell someone, "Listen to your body," I often get a jaw-dropped, blank stare in return. Most people have not been able to tune into their inner being since early childhood. No one has actually lost the ability; most have simply lost touch with it.

Start listening and soon you will be able to hear more and more. Sometimes the messages are intuitive, and will not come to the educated mind. When they come, resist the temptation to try and analyze them or you may lose them. Trust them and keep listening.

Several years ago, I was struggling with a lot of pain in my left hip and low back. One day, I drove to one of my favorite hiking spots and climbed out of my pickup truck intending to go on a nice, easy two-mile jaunt. When I started, my hip and back were hurting. Did I stop? No, I knew the walking was what I needed at that point. As I continued, the pain eased, I loosened up and I was really starting to enjoy myself. Then, less than halfway to my turnaround point, a soft internal voice whispered to me that it was time to turn back. There were no palpable physical sensations to keep me from continuing; I just knew. I was feeling strong, it was a beautiful morning, and, as tempted as I was to carry on with my hike, I turned back. My Innate Wisdom had sent me a message so I listened. As I ambled back to my truck, I began to doubt the message. I was feeling better with every step and had to fight the urge to turn back around and continue my hike. Over the years I have learned to trust intuitive messages like that when they come to me. I resisted the temptation that came from my thinking mind, and I continued back toward the parking lot. When I was within a few feet of my truck I had a sudden, screaming back spasm. I leaned up against my truck, did some deep breathing to help myself through the process, and then I did some light stretching exercises. Within a few minutes, the spasm passed. I hopped into my truck, drove home and took it easy for the rest of the day. Over the next few days my healing process accelerated. The spasm and my ability to process it— and then rest—were integral parts of my healing process. If I had ignored the subtle message that cut my hike short, I would have been a mile from the trailhead when the spasm hit me. That would have made for a slow, painful return trip and probably would have set my healing process back a few days, weeks or maybe even months. Who knows? Because I heeded the subtle message that my Innate Intelligence sent me, the hike helped my healing process instead of hindering it. I can't explain how my body knew exactly when to turn around, and I don't feel compelled to figure it out. My Innate Intelligence has a much deeper understanding of my physical body and my healing process than does my educated mind. Innate Intelligence is brilliant. Listen to it.

Work, Play and Rest

Oby had a great exercise program—life. He stayed healthy by chasing woolly mammoths, watching clouds and occasionally playing a few innings of a rough and tumble game known as rock-and-roll. Oby and his fellow cave dwellers worked, played and rested. Simple. Our modern lifestyle is much more complicated than Oby's, but this fundamental philosophy will always be valid.

Be Like Bob and Todd

Today, our friend Bob is like Todd, the gym rat. They both spend time enjoying what they love to do. Bob is the assistant team captain on the Keggler Kings; he and Terry bike at least a couple of times every week; and he makes it out fly fishing two or three weekends a month. He did have to shift his busy schedule around a bit, and the changes weren't all easy. In the end, the only real challenge was to follow through with the promises he made to himself. Now Bob sets his clock radio for 5:00 AM on fishing days, but he is usually up and already has his organic, naturally decaffeinated coffee brewing by 4:50 or so. On the days when he finds it a little bit harder to roll out of the sack, the effort is made easier by Bob's anticipation of the pleasure he will get from drifting a nymph on the sparkling waters of one of his secret fishing spots. He loves it. Awhile back he invited Todd to start coming along. Todd was excited because he had wanted to get outdoors more. He tagged along once, made a last minute excuse the next time, then never seemed to have the time after that. He would much rather go to the gym.

Now...go out and play!

Oby's Wisdom

- Oby's Two Step Fitness Program:

  1. List the physical activities you enjoy.

  2. Go out and enjoy them!

- The First Rule of Fitness: Play first!

- Do what you love and love what you do.

- Exercise is for elevating your spirit, not just your heart rate.

- By Nature, you enjoy exercise.

- Your mind can get your body off the couch.

- Listen to your body.

- Work, play, rest. It's that simple.

- Follow through on the promises you make to yourself.

- Now...really...go out and play!

Chapter Nine

Scooter's Wisdom

> *Grown men may learn from very little children,*
> *for the hearts of little children are pure, and,*
> *therefore, the Great Spirit may show to them*
> *many things which older people miss.*
> Black Elk

My good friend, Dr. Arno Burnier, tells a story of when he and his wife, Jane, were present when a friend of theirs gave birth. Shortly after the birth, when Arno and Jane were in the room with the new mother and her beautiful, healthy baby son, a nurse came in carrying a syringe full of vitamin K. In most American hospitals, newborn infants receive a vitamin K injection shortly after birth to prevent a rare bleeding disorder in infants. According to several studies, the downside of vitamin K injections—which introduce vitamin K into the newborn at 20,000 times the natural level—is that excessive levels of vitamin K may increase the risk of childhood leukemia. Arno told the nurse that the mother preferred her son not have the vitamin K injection. The nurse was rather taken aback and remarked that all babies had to have the shot. Arno pointed out: "I have a hard time believing that Nature spent nine months creating this perfect baby then slapped herself on the forehead and said, 'Oops...forgot the vitamin K.'"

You can bet Scooter never had a vitamin K injection.

Mother Nature Has a Plan

We all start out as one cell—a microscopic, fertilized egg cell. This cell divides within 24 hours and the wondrous process of human development begins. By the third day, that first cell has become 12. By day four, the cells separate into outer and inner layers, which eventually become the placenta and the embryo. During the earliest stages, all of the cells are similar to each other, yet their Innate Intelligence guides them to begin forming specific layers and cavities. They start as uniform little soldiers responding to silent commands and marching to their assigned places of duty. On about day seven, magic begins to happen. The cells begin to differentiate. In other words, new types of cells are born. A diverse mix of new cells joins our little soldiers, bringing with them countless new talents and skills. As this new life grows, the embryo becomes ever more sophisticated and complex. During the third week, the nervous system begins to form. By the end of the fourth week, the foundations of the heart, lungs, digestive system, skin, skeleton and reproductive system are in place. During the fifth week, the limbs, head and eyes begin to appear. By the end of the eighth week, all essential human characteristics are present. We now have a tiny but essentially complete human. During the remaining 30 or so weeks the baby continues to grow and mature to the point that she is capable of living on the outside.

Great plan! It has worked for billions of humans over the course of millions of years, and will remain how we come into being for as long as our species exists. Human innovation will never improve upon it.

Nature took care of even the tiniest of details. Isn't it reasonable to believe that the same brilliant Universal Intelligence that came up with this plan also mapped out what to do after birth—an equally brilliant design for the baby to grow into a vibrant, healthy, smart, spiritually-connected, emotionally-centered adult? Could it be possible that squeezing through the birth canal, suckling breast milk, crawling, falling, fevers, chicken pox, laughing, crying, playing and making mud pies may all be integral parts of the plan? Might it be possible that our scientifically designed attempts to improve on Nature are nothing more than second rate imitations?

One of the most critical areas of early childhood development is that of the spine and cranium, important not only as the central skeletal structures, but also because they house the central nervous system—the brain and spinal cord. When a baby first begins developing in the womb, the spine has one curve. By the time children reach their first birthday, their spine has four curves. Proper development of the curves is necessary for optimum skeletal and neurological functioning. The curves develop through a child's natural progression of...

lying flat...
learning to lift the head...
beginning to do shaky little baby pushups...
starting to crawl...
standing up on wobbly little legs...
taking the first steps.

Mom, Dad, family and friends marvel at every wondrous and exciting development. Each step demonstrates Nature's beautiful, incredible and brilliant plan. Unfortunately, every step of the way, many well-meaning parents unintentionally interfere. When our babies should be rolling around on the floor and starting to build strength in their arms, we have them lying on their backs in wind up swings for hours on end. The swings may be great babysitters but they deprive our growing children of necessary physical exercise. Later, when junior should be crawling around—and developing his lumbar curve—we plunk him down in a walker. As he wheels around the house, his upright position puts stress on his spine that it is not developmentally ready for. If our child is blowing out his first birthday candle and has not yet learned to walk, while the neighbors' 11 month old is already taking her first steps...well, we can't have that, can we? Mom and Dad go into high gear, trying to push their precocious progeny to perambulate. The result is unnecessary physical and emotional stress. Every child is unique and all children have their own, perfect schedules. No hurry.

Mom is Packing a Lunch

One of the most basic, important and loving choices a mother can make to help turn her baby's health inside out is to breast-feed. The Innate Wisdom of both Baby and Mom work together in synergy to create the perfect, custom tailored formula that each unique baby needs. The physical, emotional and mental benefits of breastfeeding last for a lifetime. Some of the many pluses include:

- Breastfeeding strengthens the bond between the mother and her child, enhancing family relationships.

- It provides for optimum physical, neurological, mental, emotional and social development.
- It reduces the risk of health threats ranging from sudden infant death syndrome (SIDS) and cancer, to colic and diaper rash.
- It assists in the development of maximum immune potential.

For Mom, the benefits include lower risk of such conditions as breast and ovarian cancer, depression and osteoporosis. Breastfeeding also saves time and money; you have less to buy and carry around in the baby bag. Breastfeeding also helps to save the planet. Baby formulas come in containers, which end up as waste in our landfills and on our roadsides. Manufacturing processes and preparation of the formula at home also consume precious energy resources. More information on breastfeeding is available from La Leche League International at www.LLLI.org.

Just Say No to Drugs...Starting Right Now

If Thomas Edison and Albert Einstein were children today they would both be drugged. Why? There are two reasons:
1. Because they were different, and different is often seen as a problem.
2. We have a drug for every problem.

Today's society is too attached to making children conform and fit in. Life will be better for everybody when we provide these beautiful and perfect little people a supportive and encouraging environment within which they can express their uniqueness. Kids today are different than children of past generations. Old rules no longer apply. Still, most teachers, doctors and parents persist in trying to raise, educate and care for them using methods from the past. We are trying to hammer today's round pegs into yesterday's square holes. How? With labels and drugs. If kids are different today than in the past, that must mean that something is wrong with them...right? So the appropriate corrective action is to diagnose the problem and administer the proper compound...right?

A better way

Today, far too many children are labeled as ADD or ADHD (attention deficit disorder or attention deficit hyperactivity disorder). In 2004, over 23 million prescriptions were written for drugs such as Ritalin to treat ADD and ADHD in American children. The problem with this approach is that the drugs serve only to manage the behavior of the children; they do not correct any underlying problem, cure any disease, or lead to improved cognitive functioning or learning. Our children need us to love and nurture them, not manage them.

To me, the diagnostic criteria for ADD and ADHD look pretty much the same as for what I would call AKS (active kid syndrome). On this frightening list we find such serious problems as:

- Does not listen when spoken to
- Is easily distracted
- Often fidgets or squirms
- Is constantly on the go and appears to be driven by a motor

Along with these diagnostic criteria comes the statement that they must be "severe enough to interfere with normal social and school activities." The problem is that the degree of severity is subjective. An impatient teacher with thirty kids in her classroom may find it expedient to judge a child's fidgeting and inattention as severe enough to interfere, when all the child may need is an alteration in his learning environment such as allowing him to stand up and stretch more often than the other kids. Parents can find a number of excellent books on this subject. I highly recommend *The Indigo Children* by Lee Carol and Jan Tober. I first read this book, shortly after it was published, when my son was 14 years old. As a parent, I consider it the most valuable book I ever read on raising a healthy, well-adjusted child. I wish it had been available about 15 years earlier.

Parents and teachers are beginning to understand the needs of today's children. Sadly, there are still too many who find it easier to drug their kids than to deal with them. The tragic result is that millions of today's most brilliant young minds and beautiful spirits are hidden from us by a shroud of pharmaceutical darkness. Whole foods, chiropractic care, understanding and love are better answers than drugs.

Wait a minute...back up...chiropractic?

Yes, chiropractic.

As one who has personally been through the wringer of chronic pain and disease, and has facilitated healing for people with a vast array of health challenges, I believe that life-centered chiropractic is among the most powerful healing arts on the planet. There is even a volume in the best selling *Chicken Soup for the Soul* series entitled, *Chicken Soup for the Chiropractic Soul*. Among the stories in the book are life changing miracles that have happened in the lives of all kinds of people, including many children.

Of all the people I serve, those who show the most profound improvements in their lives are teens and preteens who have had some sort of behavioral or emotional label foisted upon them. I avoid using statistics and labels—especially with kids—but if I used them, the statistic, "kids with learning disabilities or behavioral problems who have shown remarkable improvement," would approach 100%. Take, for example, a 15-year-old girl I'll call Michelle whose mother originally brought her to me because of migraine headaches. On her first visit I learned she had suffered serious, ongoing emotional trauma earlier in her life, which translated into emotional and behavioral challenges during adolescence. After several months of regular wellness care, not only were her migraines gone, but her life transformed. She told me that because of chiropractic, "I've been more confident in my life, and more happy overall. I *used to be* labeled depressed." (Italics mine.)

You can learn more about the wonders of chiropractic for children by visiting the International Chiropractic Pediatric Association website; www.ICPA4Kids.org.

Our children's gifts are our gifts. How many Edisons and Einsteins have their gifts trapped inside of themselves because we keep them drugged? Let's nurture our children in such a way that we encourage them to grow, blossom and reveal their gifts to the world.

ADD and ADHD are not the only labels that cause us to turn too quickly to chemical intervention. Every symptom, it seems, has a corresponding drug in the medicine cabinet or herb in the pantry. Fevers, sniffles and tummy aches are usually normal, healthy immune responses. Let Nature and love do the healing.

Before You Vaccinate

Whether or not to vaccinate your children is one of the most important decisions you will ever make.

Many parents today, concerned about the health and safety of their children, are electing not to vaccinate them. Contrary to what the pharmaceutical industry would have you believe, the outcry over the dangers of vaccines is not just coming from a bunch of hysterical parents. A significant portion of today's scientific and healthcare community, including prominent scientists and physicians, question the safety and effectiveness of vaccinations. Professional groups including the Association of American Physicians and Surgeons, and all of the major professional chiropractic organizations in the United States oppose mandatory childhood vaccination policies. There have even been congressional inquiries into the possible dangers of vaccinations. The U.S. Government has paid out over $2 billion in claims to vaccine-injured children and adults under the National Childhood Vaccine Injury Act of 1986. Although American children are among the most heavily vaccinated in the world, a study published in the Journal of the American Medical Association in July, 2000 comparing quality of healthcare between 13 industrialized nations, ranked the United States 13th—dead last—in infant mortality.

The vocal parents of vaccine-injured children are far from hysterical. These parents (some of whom are physicians themselves) are intelligent, well-educated, caring mothers and fathers who have done their research, and who live with the issue every day. They know what they are talking about and it behooves all of us to listen.

Consider the following: Vaccinations bypass one of the body's most critical protective systems—the skin. They contain foreign proteins that can cause adverse reactions, as well as preservatives such as mercury, aluminum, and formaldehyde that can cause significant, irreversible damage to a child's sensitive developing nervous system. Vaccinations do not provide lifelong immunity. Any immune benefit that vaccinations may provide is artificial, and not a lasting, natural immunity. Vaccinations may even be leading to an increase in certain diseases. Science is beginning to show that childhood diseases such as chicken pox may be an important part of immune system development. Preventing these diseases may actually lead to an increased risk of asthma, allergies and other conditions. Other credible scientific evidence suggests a possible link between vaccinations and brain inflammation which can lead to autism.

Many informative books and articles are available to parents who want to learn more. The best place to start is the National Vaccine Information Center web site, www.NVIC.org.

Nature didn't slap herself on the forehead and say, "Darn! Forgot the antibodies." Scooter and countless generations of troglodyte toddlers managed to grow and thrive without vaccinations.

My intent here is not to advocate a particular course of action. True, I'm primarily addressing one side of the issue. My reason for doing so is because it is *critical* to give a voice to the side of the issue that falls outside of today's deeply entrenched and highly funded conventional thinking.

This is an area where passions run deep and belief systems—on both sides—tend to be unbending. Don't take your medical doctor's, your alternative practitioner's or my word as the bottom line. On this issue, more than any other, it is important to do your own, open minded, balanced research and arrive at your own decision.

Whatever your decision, remember this:

Chemists will never match the perfection of nature.

Get Dirty!

When my son was in elementary school, I helped coach his baseball team, the Bulldogs. Our players were younger, smaller and less experienced than the players on the other teams so everyone expected us to finish in last place. But what these kids lacked in size and experience they more than made up for in spirit, determination and heart. They were scrappy, they played hard and they had a blast. After the first few practices, a team motto emerged, "Get dirty!" Parents used to joke that soon we wouldn't have a field to practice on because the players wore most of the field home with them. To everybody's amazement, except ours, we finished the season as one of the best teams in the league. At the end of the season the players presented me with two autographed baseballs. On one were penned the words, "Coach Cochran, Get Dirty!" It was signed by Maury Wills who used to play for the Los Angeles Dodgers, and is considered one of the greatest base runners in the history of the game. In 1962, he became the first player to steal more than 100 bases in a single season. In the process, he broke Ty Cobb's record that was almost 50 years old. Maury Wills was a guy who liked to get dirty. The second—and most important—of the two autographed baseballs was signed by all of the Bulldogs.

Getting dirty on the baseball diamond, rolling around in the grass, and being covered with wet puppy kisses, all help children build natural immunity. As kids are exposed to microbes from a variety of sources, their immune systems respond by developing a broad range of antibodies. These continuing challenges strengthen developing immune systems just as pumping iron builds six pack abs and rippling biceps on body builders.

Keeping our kids too squeaky clean can actually lead to weakened immune functioning and more health challenges. In the late 1990's, a hypothesis known as the Hygiene Hypothesis emerged which supports this point. A German health re-searcher named Dr. Erika von Mutius set out to show that children who grew up in the poorer, dirtier cities of East Germany developed more allergies than their counterparts in West Germany. When she compared the disease rates between the two countries she found the opposite. Dr. Von Mutius concluded that children in East Germany had fewer allergies *because* they were exposed more to other kids, animals...and dirt. Studies since then have shown that kids who live on farms, have pets, come from larger families or start day care at a younger age tend to have a lower incidence of asthma than other kids. Another report tells us that the more often kids catch colds during their early years, the less likely they are to develop asthma later on. (Colds are cool.) When kids are exposed to common bacteria, their immune systems are able to mature the way Nature designed them to. Their immune systems are on the front lines maintaining their edge while the immune systems of kids in overly clean environments are kicking back all day and letting themselves get soft and weak.

Of course good hygiene is important; just try not to take it too far. Teach your kids to wash their hands before meals but resist the temptation to hustle them to the sink and slather them with antibacterial soap every time they pet the neighbor's cat. Our well-intentioned attempts to shield our kids from every cootie in the neighborhood deprives them of essential opportunities to develop a robust immune system. Scooter lived his entire life with a dirty face. Yet he grew up big and strong enough to chase woolly mammoths for miles across the prairie and run away from the occasional growling grizzly bear.

So, believe it or not, even germs help turn health inside out. The next time your kids come in from playing outside, check their hands. Hopefully, they will have some dirt under their fingernails.

Just Play

Scooter loved spending his days playing with Proto and other children in the clan. Every sound, sight, smell and experience was a new lesson for Scooter. Every time he played—whether with friends, Proto, Oby and Fern, or alone— Scooter's body grew stronger, his mind sharper, his emotions more centered, his imagination more vivid and his spirit more awakened.

Playing is an intricate part of Nature's plan for children. During their earlier years, most of what children learn comes through their play. Children's play is an integral part of intellectual, emotional, physical and spiritual development. Allow children to play without too much guidance, direction or interference. Give them room for creative, unstructured play guided by their spirit and soul. Let the imagination run free. When a child gets a car that comes in a large box, what does he want to play with? The box, of course. A car is a car, albeit with many car possibilities; but in a box, a child can build a fort, travel in a time machine or embark upon any thrilling adventure he chooses. He can even race a car.

Respect your child's "imaginary" playmate. Imaginary playmates are as real to your children as this book is to you, and can be as important as anyone else in their lives. The question is, who are they? Are they entities from the spirit world that only their chosen human can see? Are they alter egos manifested from a child's own consciousness? Or are they only a figment of a child's imagination? Answer: Who cares? Your child has a friend to laugh and cry with; someone to argue and celebrate with; someone who understands and cares when no one else does. Imaginary playmates are companions and teachers that provide interaction and growth that no one else can offer. They are perfect playmates.

The Most Important Lesson

Teach your children every day: You are beautiful and perfect!

Several years ago, a concerned mother brought her preteen daughter, Maddie, to see me because she had been diagnosed with progressive scoliosis. X-rays that had been taken at a hospital showed that Maddie's spine had lateral curves greater than 40 degrees. Whenever she tried to stand for very long, she was in pain.

I told Maddie at the beginning of her first visit, "You are a being of beauty and perfection." The day after her first adjustment, Maddie was able to stand straight and tall for her entire art class, free of back pain. At the end of her second visit, my visual analysis showed her spine to be almost completely straight. After a few weeks of care Maddie had another medical appointment during which they took a new set of x-rays. After the exam, her mother called me, dismayed that Maddie's new x-rays showed 40-degree lateral curves. I do not take x-rays in my practice so I wondered if it could be possible for a visual analysis to show a relatively straight spine while forty-degree curves were lurking inside. Before Maddie's next visit, I consulted a chiropractic radiologist who told me that visual analysis and x-ray images will correlate with each other. "What you see is what you get," were the radiologist's exact words. When Maddie walked in the door I could immediately see that the curves were far more pronounced than they had been the last time she was in. After I adjusted her, the curves were again greatly reduced and Maddie continued to improve for the next few weeks. Then she went to the hospital for another scheduled medical exam and it all happened again. One day her spine was almost straight and the next, Maddie was x-rayed and again had 40-degree curves.

How can such a thing happen? It is a matter of consciousness. Remember, the mind is the matrix of all matter; what you look for, you find; what you think about, you create. I treated Maddie as a beautiful and perfect young girl, so that was what she was. At the hospital, they saw her as the poor little girl with the severe scoliosis, so that was what she became. The tragedy in this case was that the medical doctors convinced Maddie's parents that the scoliosis would continue to worsen. Without aggressive medical intervention, they said, Maddie may never be able to walk or sit normally, and might not be able to drive a car. Maddie's parents succumbed to the fear and never brought her back to see me. Not long after that I happened to run into them in town. Maddie was wearing a brace and was destined for surgery to have a steel rod attached to her spine. That was a cold knife in my heart because I knew that beautiful young girl did not need the brace or the surgery. Please understand that I am not criticizing Maddie's parents. Although fear seemed to be a key factor, I know they felt love and concern, and made the decision they thought was best for their daughter. This shows how damaging a fear-based approach to health can be. Fear turns off life.

Contrast Maddie's story with that of 15 year-old David, who had been diagnosed with progressive scoliosis and was under care at the same hospital as Maddie. From the very start, David and his entire family embraced the concept that they are all beautiful and perfect. After his first adjustment, David stood straighter and felt much better. Within a few weeks, the scoliosis was no longer visibly evident. We never discussed it after that. They came for life, not disease. After about a year and a half, David's mother told me that she had taken him to the hospital for an exam, and his x-rays no longer showed any evidence of progressive scoliosis. The doctors were amazed and told David and his mother he would not have to come back any more.

Self-image is important. This is true not only with issues such as self-esteem and self worth, but also with a person's image of themselves as a physical being. As Maddie and David show clearly, how your children think about themselves—and how you think about them—has a profound impact on their health and their lives. When it comes to health, today's society inundates us with an endless flood of messages telling us we are diseased and imperfect. We must change that message.

The Basic Truth—that we are all beings of beauty and perfection—must become a part of our collective consciousness. We can start by embracing it within ourselves, and then teach it at home, at school, in church, at the doctor's office, on TV, on the internet and everywhere else. Beauty and perfection can become a powerful new paradigm to create a society where our children grow up with a self-image as beautiful, perfect and inherently healthy. Teach your children every moment of every day: You are beautiful and perfect!

Your Children's Most Powerful Healer: Life!

The life force that we were all born with is the most powerful healer of all. In fact, life is the only healer there is. Some beautiful examples of the awesome healing capacity of Nature are the miracles that happen at the Oklahaven Children's Chiropractic Center in Oklahoma City. Oklahaven is a nonprofit center devoted to providing care to special needs children. Oklahaven's President and CEO, Dr. Bobby Doscher, is a very good friend of mine and a valued mentor. During my first year in chiropractic college, it was Dr. Bobby who first opened my eyes to the amazing power of Nature to heal even those deemed the most hopeless. She visited Palmer College and gave a presentation that touched me deeply. For an hour, she showed us before and after photos of kids she had served at Oklahaven. When they first came to her, many of the children looked almost lifeless. After a period of time—varying from one child to another—the photos showed how much more life they were expressing. Their eyes shone brighter. Faces that had been flat and dull had come to life with bright, shiny smiles.

The transformation in the lives of the children and their families is amazing. Although the children come to her with such challenges as muscular dystrophy, autism and cerebral palsy, Dr. Bobby focuses on turning health inside out, not treating disease. The children grow and thrive as a result of chiropractic adjustments, a whole food diet, fresh air, sunlight, exercise and lots of love and encouragement.

One wonderful story is that of a boy named Robert who, at age two, was diagnosed with juvenile rheumatoid arthritis. When Robert was five years old his doctors recommended he be placed on a powerful chemotherapy drug. Robert's family chose chiropractic instead. After the first adjustment, he was noticeably more comfortable when he walked. He has continued regular chiropractic adjustments, has become an award-winning pianist and earned a music scholarship to Oklahoma State University. As Robert's mother, Paula, points out, "He has a life that he chooses to lead instead of his arthritis determining what he can and can't do."

One of Dr. Bobby's most important lessons is commitment. Parents need to be committed, over the long haul, to their child's own beautiful and perfect process of healing and growth. The miracles that happen at Oklahaven do not usually happen overnight, but result from allowing the children to blossom, in their own time, and realize their glorious divine potential.

"What we expect from the parents is to believe in their child as a spiritual being; that the child has great potential. It does take time; it does take discipline. Many parents have seen this and they have worked hard towards it, and now they have whole children," says Dr. Bobby. "The lesson for all of us is simply to help our children reach their maximum potential through a natural way of life."

Love, Don't Label

Labels sometimes provide a useful framework to allow us to understand a situation, but labels limit. Do not let a label define your child regardless of whether that label happens to be "ADHD," "Indigo Child," or anything else. Every label carries its own parameters and expectations, and therefore, its own set of limitations. Rather than reducing children to a set of checklists, love all of them as unique, beautiful and perfect.

Don't Put Your Kids in a Box

Every child is a uniquely beautiful, perfect and complex expression of the Divine. Each has a special set of gifts—those they have been given and those they have to offer. Support and love all children with the understanding that their individual life process is perfect for them. Be present. The greatest gift you can give to a child is yourself. Respect their dreams and fantasies, and their curious thoughts, even if you cannot understand them. I have a good friend named Greg who has a lively and brilliant son named Dakotah. Once, when Dakotah was four years old, he and Greg came into see me for their adjustments. Dakotah looked at his father and asked, "Dad, what does lima bean coffee taste like?" Well, Greg couldn't come up with an answer to that, but he recognized that it was a valid question. It was important to Dakotah or he would never have thought to ask it.

Children's perspectives and curiosities are valid, even though they may diverge from our own. Delight in them. Structure, boundaries and stability are essential in children's lives, but it is just as important to give them plenty of room to flourish in their own, unique way. Except in the case of our children's safety and well-being, it is not up to us adults to force them into our way of thinking. They have important gifts to offer us so we need provide the space to allow those gifts to manifest themselves. We can learn much from the fresh, uncluttered, unjaded spirits of these new arrivals. The more we try to put them in a box—one that we have built without their permission or input—the more we limit them, and the more we deny ourselves the gifts they bear.

It is not our task to mold our children. Let them remain connected to their child nature as they mature. Create a safe environment to allow their own path to unfold, and let them follow it. Never try to force a child down your path and never judge what a child's path should be. As Hillary Rodham Clinton says in *It Takes a Village*: "Parenthood is not a second childhood and children are not miniature versions of our-selves. From the beginning they are individuals who must be respected for who they are and are meant to be."

Honor your children's dreams and fantasies. In our society, dreams are often not safe. Many people are naysayers, however well meaning and sensible they try to be. Your children's dreams are a manifestation of their spirit, and will grow, thrive and become real in a positive, encouraging environment.

Love is the real world. Loving your children is the most important and powerful gift you can give to allow them to achieve their maximum human potential.

Love turns health inside out.

Scooter's Wisdom

- Mother Nature has a brilliant plan.

- Creep, crawl and walk rather than swing, slouch and roll.

- Mom is packing the perfect lunch.

- Let Nature and love do the healing.

- Chemists will never match the perfection of Nature.

- Get dirty!

- Just play.

- Teach your children: You are beautiful and perfect!

- Nature is the most powerful healer.

- Don't put your kids in a box.

- Love turns health inside out.

Chapter Ten

A Day in the Life of Oby

Oby *lived!* That is what Nature had in mind.

Late one evening, our hirsute hero found himself up on the fragrant, verdant hill he so loved, lying on his back in the soft, deep clover, gazing in awe at the beauty of the heavens above. As the hot summer sun had given away to twilight, it had treated Oby to a lively and colorful light show. Now, a sparkling swath of stars was beginning to adorn the darkening sky. A gentle and comforting evening breeze brought welcome respite from the heat of the day. Oby felt happy and he loved life.

A Positive Attitude Turns Health Inside Out

Oby had risen before the sun that morning as he did every morning. Despite such modern conveniences as stone wheels and his sleek, new, ergonomically designed club—an OakLite

XL—the daily life of a cave dweller was a busy one indeed. Sometimes, he and his fellow hunters chased woolly mammoths for days at a time so that they could bring home meat for their families. Predators such as saber tooth tigers often threatened, and Oby kept a weather eye for hostile bands of cavemen. The cave people spent endless hours gathering enough fruit, nuts, berries, vegetables and firewood to keep themselves alive through the harsh winters. Then there was all of the time spent chipping away at chunks of obsidian to fashion the tools they needed. Life brought them times of plenty and times of frightening scarcity. On some days they relaxed in relative security and safety, and other times they huddled together in fear. Through the peaks and valleys of life, Oby maintained a positive, upbeat outlook. Oby understood that it was up to him to choose his attitude. He chose a happy, optimistic way of being. Of course, Oby was human. He had a full range of emotions and, like anyone else; he sometimes felt anger, sadness, despair, fear and frustration. When these feelings welled up, he acknowledged them, learned from them and moved on. He never tried to suppress or deny them; he just chose not to dwell on them or allow his feelings to anchor him in the past. For Oby, living positively did not mean going through life with a painted-on smile and an artificial cheeriness. He understood that he could keep a generally positive outlook even when life's inevitable curveballs challenged him.

Many of the other cave dwellers shared Oby's sunny outlook on life. They felt that living with a positive attitude was healthier and more productive than wallowing in their woes. As he marveled at the Milky Way emerging above him, Oby's thoughts drifted back to a hunting trip a couple of months earlier. As he and a hunting party had pursued two elusive woolly mammoths, they had encountered more difficulty than usual. Some of his band had become despondent. They were angry at life, at each other and even angry at the mammoths themselves. How rational was that? They whimpered about the danger, the drudgery, the weather and everything else. They whined about all of the time they had to spend away from their families, and then later on, they complained about their families. In short, they went through this experience as they did the rest of their lives—as helpless victims. Oby thought of these people as, *"the Negatives."*

Others, like Oby and his closest friends, took a different approach. Destiny had dealt them the exact same hand as the Negatives, but these guys were diggin' life. Oby never thought of mammoth chasing as drudgery. He loved his work. Oh sure, it was hard, and it could be frustrating and dangerous at times, but every day promised fresh excitement. He remembered the day when the uncooperative pair of mammoths seemed to disappear into the ether. Oby and his friends were hot, tired and hungry, and at a loss over what to do. Instead of groaning about the lost mammoths, they got together, assessed their strategy and formulated a better course of action for the next day. They chose to move forward with optimism and confidence rather than look backward in anger and frustration. After agreeing on their new plan, they gathered for their meal and shared funny stories from their latest pursuit of the wily Pleistocene pachyderms. Oby chuckled as he recalled a story his friend, Harry, had told of how he had been crawling through the grass when a large spider suddenly scampered across his nose. It was amazing, Harry had shared, how quickly priorities could change from mammoths to spiders. Later, their conversation turned to amusing stories about their children. Then silence fell upon them as the distant mountains became a canvas on which the setting sun painted a dancing masterpiece in hues of orange, red and purple. For some of those who were outside of Oby's group of friends, it had been a miserable day. For Oby, the events of the day had generated great memories that he would enjoy for years to come.

The life you live comes from within you, and not from external circumstances. The radiant sun of a positive attitude begins to rise within you as soon as you make the choice that positive is the way you will be. As your inner sun continues to rise and bring light and warmth to your life, it reveals the glimmering luster of the jewels that lie within you.

Playing Turns Health Inside Out

The bewitching call of an owl pulled Oby back to the present moment. Oby felt tired, but it was a good tired. After endless days of hard work, his band had stored a lot of meat, fruit, nuts, vegetables and firewood for the coming winter. Much work still lay ahead, but the time had come for a breather. Even our ancient ancestors knew that life was not all about work. If they just kept grinding away, then work would become drudgery, and they would ultimately be less efficient and get less work done. In fact, if they did not take a play break now and then, every part of their lives would take a downhill turn. As one of Oby's friends had chuckled, "all work and no play makes Oby a dull boy." So today, Oby and his friends got together for a rousing game of rock-and-roll. The game entailed one player throwing a small rock as hard as he could to another player who would then try to whack it out of the meadow with his club. The game always included a lot of running, laughing, shouting and rolling around in the dirt.

Rock-and-roll was fun. Oby was not the strongest or fastest player, but he always played with more heart, spirit and gusto than anybody else. Hence his nickname, "The Obynator." He played hard, he got dirty and he had fun doing it. A raucous game of rock-and-roll enlivened him.

Love Turns Health Inside Out

A slender crescent moon began to peek above the shadowy prairie and Oby knew it was starting to get late. He wanted to get back to Fern and Scooter before Scooter went to sleep. Oby loved Fern and Scooter; they brought more joy into his life than anything else. His work kept him away from the home fires for many days at a time, so he made it a point to be with them as much as he could. In fact, Oby had taken them along to his rock-and-roll game today. Scooter had a grand time crawling around and trying to whack tiny rocks with a small stick. Oby chuckled at Scooter even more than whacking and chasing rocks himself. Scooter was cool. When Oby got home, Scooter squealed with joy and crawled as quickly as he could to his dad. Oby and Fern spent the next hour or so quietly playing with Scooter until his eyes began to droop. After Scooter was asleep, Fern and Oby spent some quiet time reflecting on the day, sharing dreams about the future and enjoying one another.

Oby and Fern's relationship was not all fun and games. They had their conflicts from time to time, just like everyone else. When disagreements arose, they worked through them together and they grew with every challenge. The love that Oby shared with Fern enlivened him and brightened his life. He was not concerned with what he could get out of the relationship. He just loved Fern. Was she perfect? Well, if Oby had wanted to, he could have grumbled about Fern's shortcomings. What would have been the point of that? His complaints would have been nothing more than his own judgments. Oby understood the divine truth that Fern was beautiful and perfect.

Oby innately knew that love was the most powerful force in the universe, and the more he could love—Fern, Scooter, his family, his friends, people who did not like him, people he did not even know, the gifts of Nature, life itself—the stronger and healthier he would be. Oby just loved.

Not all of Oby's friends had mates. A few were frustrated and disappointed that they had no one special to share their life with. Others chose to be more positive, knowing that no matter what, they could always love. To them, love was not a thing, but a choice they made, and a way of being that they actively nurtured. Parents, brothers and sisters, pets, friends, life...there were so many ways to love. They had abundant love to share and they shared it generously. They wove glowing strands of love into the matrix and in so doing, attracted love into their lives. Although none of them had ever heard of Mother Teresa, they embodied her lesson; "Love is a fruit in season at all times, and within reach of every hand." Like Oby, they just loved.

Exercising the Mind Turns Health Inside Out

Oby thought a lot about love. In fact he thought about all kinds of things. Of course, he did not have any books to read. The earliest scholars had not even carved their wisdom onto the first clay tablets. Oby studied and pondered the lessons of Nature. The point was not to accumulate vast quantities of new information, but to stimulate and exercise his mind. As we know, "The mind is the matrix of all matter."

There was so much to learn and discover. For example, Oby observed that in the years with the most lightning during the spring storms, the grass grew taller and thicker, and the woolly mammoths fatter. True, it was a brilliant insight, but more important was the growth of the mind. As Oby's mind grew and his intelligence deepened, he enabled others to do the same. He was connected to everyone and everything else, and by pondering, thinking and stimulating his own mind, he was expanding the collective consciousness of humanity. But...it was important for Oby not to let his thinking mind get in the way of the Innate Wisdom with which he had been endowed. As Albert Einstein would remind Oby's descendants one day in the distant future: "The intuitive mind is a sacred gift and the rational mind is a faithful servant. We have created a society that honors the servant and has forgotten the gift." As long as Oby remembered the difference between the sacred gift and the servant, his mind would be a powerful force for turning his health inside out.

Relaxation, Peace and Quiet Turn Health Inside Out

Whew! So much working, playing, loving and thinking. Oby knew that it was also important to kick back, relax and recharge when he could. That was why he made it a point to spend quiet moments with Fern and Scooter as often as possible. Peace and quiet drew Oby to his hilltop every day. Lying in the soft clover and watching the clouds gave Oby a perfect space for reflection, meditation, connection with Spirit and soothing his soul.

Life is an art, not an act.

Oby's Wisdom

- Live!

- Be positive.

- Play.

- Love.

- Think.

- Kick back.

- Life is an art, not an act.

Afterword

> *If you want to build a ship, don't herd people together to collect wood, and don't assign them tasks and work but rather, teach them to long for the endless immensity of the sea.*
> Antoine de Saint-Exupery

Oby's simple wisdom is not about collecting materials and performing tasks; rather, I hope this book stirs within you a longing to spend your life exploring the vast and bottomless sea of human potential that lies, mysterious and welcoming, within you.

Make a Commitment to Life for Life

I ask you to make one commitment: a lifelong commitment to your own potential. Health and well-being are a lifelong synergy of spirit and action, and not just a list of goals, statistics and achievements. Progress and results are only judgments, especially when you attach them to a timeline. Trying to judge or predict your potential will limit you. The commitment is what is important.

Lifelong commitments have their ups and downs. You will enjoy times of laser focus and unwavering will. There will also be stretches—some long, some short—when you slip. Recognize slippage as an opportunity to learn and grow. When you feel yourself edging a bit too close to a slippery slope or even if you start sliding headlong down it, you can pick up this book and reread the chapters that apply to the challenges you face. Then recommit yourself to Oby's simple wisdom as your guiding inspiration.

Listen to Your Inner Cave Dweller

There will be days when you wander back into the confusing fog of our complex society. Best-selling authors, eloquent speakers, sensible doctors, and well-meaning family and friends will bury you under heaps of brilliant, scientifically sound—and often bad—advice. You may not know where to turn. In those times, remember that the human design that we consider high tech will never match the simple, elegant genius of Nature. Nature's simple plan always works. When your educated mind is at a loss as to which high tech route to try, be guided by the decisions that Oby did not have to make. Instead of fretting over which nutritional supplements are the best for you, go buy some locally grown organic spinach. Rather than stress out about trying to make it to the gym three times this week, go out and play. Oby's simple wisdom is your lighthouse in the fog.

Before You Can Do, You Must Be

Any successful enterprise requires effort—doing. That said, your doing must be built upon a foundation of being. Where you end up in life is driven more by who you are than by what you do. Without a rock solid foundation, your mansion will topple.

This book is not a litany of rules but a set of simple guiding principles. Following them will empower you to lay a foundation on which you can build a life glowing with love, joy and vibrant health. Oby does not have a one-size-fits-all program to offer. If you want to commit to a structured program, go for it, but be sure to build your program on the firm foundation of Oby's simple wisdom. Then, if you waver in your commitment to the program, you will still be standing on solid ground.

That which you seek already exists inside of you, just as the symphonies of the future are already contained within the matrix. The composer, conductor and musician do not create symphonies; they reveal them. Your task is to reveal you. It is what you do that makes things happen, but it is who you are that determines what happens.

Empower Your Potential, Not Your Problems

Today's healthcare system concerns itself almost exclusively with intervention. We devote almost all of our time, money and energy to symptoms and disease, or their underlying causes. You are whole, vibrant, beautiful and perfect, and not just a collection of problems. First and foremost, follow your Doctor Within; make *turning your health inside out* your primary approach to health.

Nature is Timeless

The details of human existence vary over the course of lifetimes and generations but the fundamental laws of Nature remain unchanged. Your educated mind has no idea where your journey will end up taking you. Only Spirit knows. Any goal, any plan, any expectation, desire, or vision that you may hold for the future, is tiny compared to the undiscovered gifts that you already own.

Pursuing a vision and planning for the future can be useful and important, but the final masterpiece is always different from the one you beheld in your mind's eye when your paintbrush made its first bold strokes upon the canvas of your life. Your path will diverge to beautiful vistas you could not have imagined, by way of dark canyons you never expected. The future is uncertain and ever changing. Do not allow fear of the unknown to keep you from doing what is right in this moment. Ralph Waldo Emerson gave us some sage advice when he so eloquently stated, "The right performance of this hour's duties will be the best preparation for the hours and ages that follow it."

The timeless and universal principles of Nature are always your best guide in the performance of this hour's duties. The clouds you watch today serve the same important purpose and are just as beautiful to behold as those Oby enjoyed so many generations ago. Embracing the simple yet powerful gifts of Nature will lead you down the path of living—really living—a life of joy, abundance, love, fulfillment and vibrant health.

Oby's Wisdom

- Make one commitment: a lifelong commitment to your own potential.

- Don't judge your potential; just maximize it.

- Commit to life for life.

- The human design that we consider high tech will never match the simple, elegant genius of Nature.

- What you do makes things happen; who you are determines what happens.

- Empower your potential, not your problems.

- First and foremost, follow your Doctor Within.

- The genius of Nature is timeless.

- The timeless and universal principles of Nature will lead you down the path of love, fulfillment, happiness, peace and vibrant health.

About the Author

Dr. Mark William Cochran

Mark William Cochran is a doctor who has walked the healing path himself. His visionary philosophy and passion for life have grown from his experiences as a healer and from journeying with health challenges of his own.

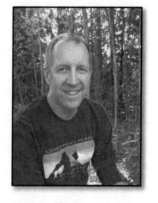

Mark's unique and gentle approach to healing calls upon ancient spiritual healing concepts to help awaken each person's own natural potential for vibrant health. He is a living testimonial to the power of his own healing approach. For many years, the pain of inflammatory arthritis made it a painful challenge for him to climb just one flight of stairs. At age 47, Mark experienced a quantum shift in his health and at 49, ran his first marathon.

Mark's walk on the healing path has not only been physical, but also a journey of the soul. In 2000, while on a chiropractic mission trip to India, Mark received a beautiful revelation that has since become the foundation of his philosophy as a healing facilitator. On one especially long day in a remote farming community, unable to communicate verbally with the people he was serving, he found himself mentally conveying a simple message to each of them: *"You are a being of beauty and perfection."*

"Since that incredible moment in India, that has been my most important message to every person I serve. From that starting point, we work in synergy to reveal the light and life that glows within everybody as their deepest, truest essence. This simple and empowering truth changes lives."

Of his many years in pain, Mark remembers, "I tried *everything*. And I've learned that what serves us best is simple. Spirit has already given us the most important and powerful gift—*life*. Growing, healing and thriving happen when we reconnect with our core essence and express the vitality within."

Mark's miraculous healing story has been chronicled in two notable inspirational books: *A Book of Miracles; Inspiring True Stories of Healing, Gratitude and Love* by Dr. Bernie S. Siegel and *Thank God I...Volume Three; Triumph Through Tragedy* created by John Castagnini.

Lovers of Nature and the great outdoors, Mark, his lovely wife, Cricket and their fuzzy feline companions, Magick and Angel, feel blessed to live, love, work and play amid the towering pines, majestic mountains and sparkling lakes of the Idaho panhandle.

The End?

No. Just the Beginning...!

> *There must be a beginning of any great matter,*
> *but continuing unto the end, until it be thoroughly finished,*
> *yields the true glory.*
> **Sir Francis Drake**

Thank you for purchasing *Oby's Wisdom! A Caveman's Simple Guide to Health and Well-being*. And congratulations on taking this important step toward *turning your health inside out!*

Finishing this book is not an ending, but the beginning of an exciting new journey for you. To show my appreciation to you for buying *Oby's Wisdom*, I have put together an entertaining free video action guide to help you incorporate Oby's most important lessons into your full and eventful life.

Go to the link below and sign up to have the action guide delivered directly to you by email.

www.DrMarks-Holistic-Health.com/oby-action-guide.html

Book Clubs...

Reading Groups...

> *Each friend represents a world in us, a world not born until they arrive, and it is only by this meeting that a new world is born.*
> Anais Nin

Discovering greater levels of health and well-being...what better way for friends to help friends birth new worlds from within?

Oby's Wisdom is an inspiring and thought provoking book for your book club or reading group to study, discuss, ponder...and grow from!

Go to the link below to download a free reading guide.

www.DrMarks-Holistic-Health.com/oby-reading-guide.html

CPSIA information can be obtained at www.ICGtesting.com
Printed in the USA
BVOW07s0527270215

389471BV00001B/6/P